The

FATAL LINK

THE CONNECTION BETWEEN SCHOOL SHOOTERS AND THE BRAIN DAMAGE FROM PRENATAL EXPOSURE TO ALCOHOL

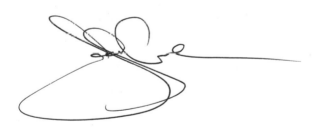

Jody Allen Crowe

Outskirts Press, Inc.
Denver, Colorado

Outskirts Press, Inc.
http://www.outskirtspress.com

ISBN: 978-1-4327-2917-2

Library of Congress Control Number: 2008938469

Outskirts Press and the "OP" logo are trademarks belonging to Outskirts Press, Inc.

PRINTED IN THE UNITED STATES OF AMERICA

The Author

Jody Allen Crowe began his career in education on one of the reservations in northern Minnesota. As a teacher and the School Effectiveness Team Facilitator for the Bug-O-Nay-Ge-Shig School, he designed and implemented a middle school that was awarded the Blue Ribbon School Award from President Clinton. He moved to the Mille Lac Band of Ojibwe as the first full time principal of the first school in the nation built with casino revenues. There, as the Nay Ah Shing School Early Childhood, K-12 principal, he led the school to the 2002 National Indian School Board Association 4 C's Award, recognized as the school of the year award for the 184 Bureau of Indian Education schools. While at Nay Ah Shing School, he designed and implemented an Ojibwe Language program that was awarded the John F. Kennedy Harvard School of Business Award High Honors designation. He has designed and implemented two highly effective Intensive Services Programs for Emotional and Behaviorally Disabled students in two different states on two different reservations. He served for two years as superintendent of the Shoshone Bannock School in Fort Hall, Idaho.

For three years, Crowe consulted with tribal schools, writing grants, designing program and curriculum, providing interim administration for tribal schools doing principal searches and consulting with the National Indian School Board Association in the Creating Sacred Places for Children Initiative. His experiences have taken him to six different reservations in four different states.

Crowe moved from Indian education into public school education in 2007. He was the Director of TEAM Academy Charter School in southern Minnesota for two years.

Crowe has served on the Principal's Advisory Committee to the National Board for Professional Teaching Standards. He was selected for the prestigious Bush Educators Program in the state of Minnesota, where, for two years, he studied Educational Leadership under the tutelage of professors from Stanford, Harvard, University of Michigan, University of Chicago, and the University of Minnesota. He holds a Bachelor of Science in Elementary Education from Bemidji State University, a Masters of Science in Public School Administration from Bemidji State University, and is an alumnus of the Sixth Year Licensure Program from the University of St. Thomas in St. Paul, MN. He holds superintendent, principal, elementary and middle school math teacher certifications in the state of Minnesota.

Jody Allen Crowe founded and serves as Executive Director of Healthy Brains for Children, a non-profit charitable organization with a mission of stopping prenatal exposure to alcohol. This organization develops and trains Healthy Brains for Children chapters in communities worldwide with a singular focus on this important mission. Information to start a chapter in your community can be found at www.healthybrainsforchildren.org.

Acknowledgements

I want to first thank my family. I chose a road less traveled in my occupation and my family were the ones who had to live with my choice. To my wife and children, thank you. JoLynn, thank you for our 31 years, even though the last year was mainly me staring at a computer screen. Jared, thank you for giving me inspiration as you served our country in Iraq. Jessica, Lucas, Katiya and Ian, you kept my spirits up the entire time I was away from the family while in Idaho. Jace, thank you for the memories of the days we drove to Nay Ah Shing School together and for your inner drive to be the best you can be.

Many people helped in the writing of this book. I have worked with many teachers over my eighteen years on reservations. Every one of you deserves a huge thank you for your commitment to your students. Several deserve mention. Thank you Judy for being a colleague who has been so supportive since our years co-teaching in the portable classrooms. Your help with editing was much appreciated. Thank you Jon for the support while I was away from my family. I look forward to working with you in the future. Thank you Janet for your openness to learning about FASD and your support of Healthy Brains for Children. Thank you Jerry Negen and the Crow Wing County Jail staff for allowing me to survey the inmates. Your willingness and support is greatly appreciated.

Others who believe in what I have to say deserve thanks. Peter, a longtime friend helped me focus on what I needed to do. Thank you, Peter, for the years of friendship and support. Chris, a Grand Rapids classmate, volunteered to read and critique my manuscript. Thank you for taking the time and for the editing. I started this project after working with Bill Lawrence of the *Ojibwe News* on an editorial on FAS. Thank you, Bill, for giving a jumpstart on this project. As this project developed, I met Roxanne Jensen, a former North Dakota State Representative. She was instrumental in the developmental editing of the manuscript. Thank you, Roxanne, so very much for your insights and support.

To the relatives of the school shooters who will remain unnamed, thank you for taking the time to visit with me. Thank you for your willingness to find and speak the truth about the mother of the shooter. Your contribution to this study is immeasurable.

A grateful thank you to Larry Oakes and the editors of the Minneapolis Star Tribune who challenged me to make this a stronger book. Your insistence of a higher standard makes the message that much stronger.

Thank you to all the students I have worked with over the years. I will always take with me the good times. I learned tremendously while working with you. Now I am giving what I learned to others.

Table of Contents

Foreword

The book you are about to read is revolutionary. Our nation is suffering a national epidemic called Fetal Alcohol Spectrum Disorder (FASD.) It may be affecting one quarter of our citizens. The amazing and disturbing part of this epidemic is that it is preventable, yet mostly overlooked. FASD is the most avoidable type of mental retardation.

Alcohol consumption by a mother during pregnancy has a direct link to fetal brain damage. The destruction to the fetus' neurological system is more dangerous than crack, meth or cocaine to the baby. The resulting damage has led to behavioral disorders ranging from ADHD to autism to gang activity to high school shooting massacres. How can the idea of "No Child Left Behind" be successful if the tools needed to "learn" are missing from the brains of our children?

Also, the resulting cost to our nation is staggering. Our medical, judicial/correctional systems, educational responsibilities and social services bear the weight of paying our money to handle this preventable epidemic.

Unfortunately our medical, psychological, educational, and law enforcement sources are generally oblivious to understanding FASD. Our 21st century lifestyle supports and condones alcoholic drinking. Sometimes pregnant women are even encouraged to have a drink once in a while to help with relaxation by their doctor. Beer, liquor, and wine are a normal facet of our society. Used at the wrong time, however, a fetus becomes a victim.

Jody Allen Crowe provides a fascinating, timely, insightful, but shocking presentation on how FASD should be recognized and prevented. It is amazing that this epidemic has been so poorly understood.

By the time you put this book down you'll have a clear understanding of a problem that is changing our society for the worse. Yet prevention of FASD needs only one thing – stop the drinking during pregnancy. "Bravo!" for Mr. Crowe's beacon of light.

Peter Johnson
Healthy Brains for Children

CHAPTER One
That Day in October 1966

"Two people have been shot at the High School!" Any lesson plans for October 5, 1966, went by the wayside as the teachers in Grand Rapids School District 318 heard the news.

I clearly remember the day. My fifth grade teacher was getting reports of a shooting at the high school. Terror reigned. Our tranquil little town had been traumatized by an unthinkable act of violence. A teacher and a student were shot. A local cop was the hero who took the gun away from the shooter. Throughout the morning the story changed and grew into a full shootout. Stories circulated that he was shooting in the hallway when the administrator walked out and was shot, wait, no, he was outside shooting and hit the other student and the administrator got in the way. On and on, the story morphed. We were hearing there was a confrontation between the police and the shooter and he hid behind some logs and was shooting at the cops. We heard the cops had to physically disarm him. We went home that night to our families and compared stories. Some wondered if this kid in our town was in any way copying the tragic Bell Tower massacre in Austin, Texas, two months prior.

Our little northern Minnesota town, nestled on the banks of the Mississippi surrounded by pristine lakes and tall forests, had just experienced the first of Minnesota's school shootings and one of the first school shooting in the nation. Grand Rapids High School, where generations of kids from all walks of life mingled, had forever been changed. There were no satellite trucks, no live feeds to the world, no reporters camped out in front of the victims' houses, no in-depth interviews with students who witnessed the shooting, no video of students running from the school in panic. All we had was the local twice-a-week newspaper writing a couple of articles detailing the events of the day. Our school quickly returned to normal, as much as could be expected after this totally unexpected and out of the ordinary event.

Eight days after the shooting, Mr. Forrest L. Willey, the courageous administrator, died of his wounds. He had bravely stood in front of the shooter and asked for the gun, upon which the shooter fired three shots at him, hitting him twice. The student victim, who had been critically wounded by a shot in the chest, survived. As the news of this tragic event spread, the shooter was identified. He quickly became the target of vicious rumors and gossip. He was painted as this violent, weird, strange acting, deviant kid who, of course, after the fact, was certainly capable of such violence. Stories spread about how he was picked on and how he had brought bullets to school warning others that the bullets were the ones that would kill them. Students who rode on his bus talked about his "different" behavior. His family was dragged through the same mud. His behaviors were blamed on the parenting ability of his parents, and, by now, everyone knew there was something wrong in the family. How could they bring up such a child?

Due to the stories I heard, I had this vision of a short, fat, black haired, pimply kid bringing a gun to school and shooting one of the "good" kids. His sister was ostracized for the remainder of her high school life. He was sentenced and adjudicated to the legal system, leaving the system when he was 21 years old. Grand Rapids lost track of him.

The town folk moved on, with most putting that day far into the recesses of their mind, until another school shooter on some distant campus broke open the long forgotten memories. The Grand Rapids story remained a local story until the student victim broke his silence and spoke about the lifetime of regret he experienced after the shooting. The memories were still there. The seconds of gunfire in the outdoor common area of the Grand Rapids Junior and Senior High School left a lifetime of painful, regretful memories.

Eight years after the shooting, our classmates honored two other graduates and me by selecting us to receive the "Forrest L. Willey Good Citizenship Award." Little did I know at that time, the memory of Mr. Willey would be a driving force in my life. The little paper certificate continues to grace my office wall reminding me of the honor.

After many years as a school administrator, I looked back and found I had been in similar situations as Mr. Willey. I felt a strong bond to him as I began the research on school shooters. Many times I visualized myself acting in a similar fashion, and in three situations stepped up to students with what were thought to be real guns and several times taking knives from students in order to protect other students and adults in the school. As I write this book, I feel I am able to provide some answers to why that shooting happened that October day in Grand Rapids, when Minnesota experienced its first school shooter and how that shooting is linked with school shootings across the nation.

CHAPTER TWO
My Journey

I was abruptly awakened by the sound of the phone at 11:45 p.m. on a rather normal Thursday night. The lateness of the call and the tone of Brad's voice shook me into sudden alertness.

"I just received a call from the Mille Lacs County Sheriff's Department." Those words started a weekend of chaos and mayhem at Nay Ah Shing School and in the Mille Lacs community in central Minnesota. The fragile truce with normalcy was shaken to its foundations. Only time would tell if the destruction that night would serve to strike down the advances of the last two years or serve to draw the students into a greater determination to create a better world for their community.

In the mid 1990's, the Mille Lacs Band of Ojibwe prided themselves on the accomplishments of their people. Two new casinos, pumping millions of dollars into the government coffers, enabled the Band to build an infrastructure second to none on Minnesota's reservations. Two schools made up the centerpieces of the infrastructure, schools that housed children from infants through 12th grade. These schools were the pride of the community, watched

5

over with jealous pride by neighbors during after school hours and weekends to ensure that what happened to the other structures in the community over the years did not happen to the new schools.

Two years prior to the late night call, in November of 1993, I took the job of principal of the Nay Ah Shing Schools. I walked into new school buildings that did not have the systems in place to support a school. Students roamed the building and grounds at will, challenging teachers and each other whenever the chance presented itself. Fights and verbal insults were daily, if not hourly, events. Teachers locked themselves into their rooms to stay away from students. Students did not trust teachers. Teachers did not trust students. I was looked upon as someone who had experience with building a successful school program and who would do the same at Nay Ah Shing. I gave myself five years to create a safe and supportive atmosphere in which students could thrive academically and socially, and if not, I was not the man for the job.

"Someone broke into the school and trashed it." Brad, the Auxiliary Services Director, said and informed me that he was on his way to the school.

"I'll be right there."

I dressed and broke the speed limit traveling the 30 miles to the school over straight country roads after midnight. Walking up to the school, I could see piles of glass covering the front entrance, chairs tipped over, and the front display of traditional clothing on a mannequin crumpled on the floor, covered with glass. Brad was beginning the cleanup as I looked around, trying to conceal how upset I was on seeing the violation of our school.

On further inspection of the building, we found the window used as an entrance, the rock used to shatter the double plate glass, and the room that was trashed first. The TV and cart were thrown on the floor, along with a video camera, a computer monitor, and notebooks and paper in malicious abandonment. The intruders had broken into the In-School Suspension room. The intruders moved to the gymnasium where fire extinguishers were shot off, creating a coating of dust in which shoe prints were left, on to the hallways and into the front office, where a large plate glass window was battered in to gain entrance to the office proper. A keyboard was destroyed, two chairs were damaged, and a door was battered by two fire extinguishers, which were thrown on the floor. As I surveyed the damage using a video camera, a sense of being violated washed over me, and for the first time I can remember, I felt defeated.

Five hours of clean up allowed us to hold school the next morning. The students were upset with the condition of the school. I had conversations with the staff and asked them to shape their conversations with the students concerning the damage, focusing on how the damage was directed at them and their possession, the school. High School Seniors voiced their feelings to the Middle School students, creating a positive interaction and learning experience for all of us. I left the school before noon, tired, but encouraged by the students.

Little did I know, as I tried to sleep that afternoon, that what I had witnessed the previous 16 hours was only the beginning. The shattered window had seemingly opened the school to the abnormality of the community, and our students were sucked into the patterns of behavior that permeated the village. Why was this community in such disarray?

On the following Monday, I was met at the door with a myriad of incidents that had happened in our school since I had left for the weekend. A theft of a computer and tapes from the Superintendent's office, a fight between two bus drivers leaving one with injuries that disabled him for three weeks, a custodian on a binge, a student who threatened to "take out" teachers as he tapped a bullet on his desk, and students who ran away from a long distance high school field trip the previous Friday after I had left the school all came at me in rapid succession.

As these reports hit me from every angle, my mind drifted back to a previous time and place where thirty-five students from another tribal school, the Bug-O-Nay-Ge-Shig School in northern Minnesota, were lined up to step on the bus in St. Paul. I frantically ran through the Minnesota Science Museum looking for three girls who had been with us only minutes before. They were nowhere to be seen, and an hour later I was in the St. Paul Police Department filing a missing children's report after the unsuccessful search for the girls. Hours later and three students short, the other teachers and I were explaining to parents and the superintendent. I should have been prepared and expecting something to happen, but my lack of experience in dealing with the abnormal behaviors led me to be rather naive about what students would do if given the chance. Fortunately, the three were found within a week.

When I was considering the job at Nay Ah Shing on the Mille Lacs Reservation, my colleagues informed me that the Mille Lacs Reservation was very traditional, but had a high incidence of alcohol abuse. While teaching on the Leech Lake Reservation, I had two students from the Mille Lacs area who were in a foster home on the Leech Lake reservation. They would occasionally visit their mother and return in rough shape emotionally, knowing that their mother was not ready to regain custody of them. Both boys were Special Education students with a label of Specific Learning Disabilities (SLD) and Emotional Behavioral Disabilities (EBD). Both boys were hard to handle and had little ability to cope with changes in their lives. Both boys had few social skills. Their behaviors were no different than a majority of students in my classroom and in the school, but with these two boys, I had more information about the use of alcohol by their mother, provided to me by their foster mother.

I assumed their behaviors were a result of the displacement and current alcohol use by their mother. Once again, I was naïve in what I assumed. As a new teacher, I was experiencing many aberrant behaviors and saw many students with physical deformities. Students had nicknames referencing their almond shaped eyes, a trait shown by many students in the school. One student had to have his rectum rebuilt, had other physical deformities, had significant behavioral problems, and was low academically and had the same "look."

Another student attached himself to the adults at the school because the other students targeted him. This student was very low academically, had the same "look" about him, and was incompetent to take care of himself, as evidenced by the time I was asked by the fifth grade female teacher to take him out of the classroom to see if he had soiled himself. He continued to deny that he had, even when I took him into the bathroom and struggled through the stench as I cleaned him, one paper towel at a time, from his buttocks to his ankles, both legs. He was not the least bit embarrassed nor did he show any concern as to what others thought of him soiling his clothes, a seemingly total lack of social awareness.

At that time, I didn't know that trait was an indication of

something much more debilitating than a different outward appearance. So many students were unable to read and write. More had behavioral difficulties. Some were violent. Some could change the environment of the school just by being there. Many were promiscuous. Suicides were prevalent. Some were predators, others were very vulnerable. It seemed as if the statistics were turned upside down. Instead of having the majority of the students functioning at their chronological age and a few having a difficult time, I was experiencing the majority of my students having a difficult time, with few functioning at or possibly near their chronological age. Many, if not most, students lived with grandmothers, aunts, or in foster care. Sexual deviancy was evident, continually displayed by the student's behaviors and through the tragic stories we heard. The impact of brain damage from alcohol was evident in their social behaviors, their academic behaviors, and in their physical characteristics, but I did not have a clue that what I was seeing was evidence of prenatal exposure to alcohol.

Throughout my years at my first school, I was sucker punched in the face, had my glasses broken twice, was punched in the ear, and was bull-rushed by two students who tried to get out of my classroom, and these incidents were with 6th grade and younger students. I stopped more fights that I can count and witnessed explosive anger, retaliation, remorse, and an unsettling lack of conscience - a place where the abnormal had become normal.

One day in my first year of teaching, while working with a student in the middle of the room, I looked up to see one of my most disruptive students attack another student, who happened to be an instigator. By the time I got to them, the larger of the two had taken the other to the ground and was pummeling him with his fists. I grabbed the attacker, put him in a bear hug and pulled him off the smaller student. We both fell to the ground. The other students were gathering around, watching this unfold in the front of the classroom. I did not have any way of alerting others for help, other than to send a student to the office. I yelled to one of the trusted students to run for help as I held the attacker to the floor.

The lesson I learned at that moment has followed me throughout my career. My actions to break up the fight put both myself and the student I was restraining in danger. The smaller student, who had jumped to his feet, had a clear shot at the attacker's head. I could hear the sickening thud as the smaller student kicked his attacker full in the face while I held him in a bear hug. Fortunately, help arrived and neither student was seriously injured in the melee. Both of these students fit the profile of FASD and went on to have seriously disrupted school experiences, heavy gang involvement, one was shot and wounded in a gang incident, and both were incarcerated throughout most of their late teenage and early adult years.

The first time I looked into totally empty eyes was my first year of teaching and it has never left my memory. This sixth grade student had enrolled in school midway through the year. He had not made it past the midway mark in the resident school district, a fact not lost on me when I looked at his record. He was nowhere near grade level in achievement, and had a litany of behavioral issues from his prior school. This was not unique in the Bug-O-Nay-Ge-Shig School, as many students open enrolled to our school when the going got tough in the public schools.

He came to me before I knew about FASD. I had eight EBD students in the room who eventually qualified for special education the following year when a licensed EBD teacher was hired. Adding one more difficult student to the mix stressed my patience and capabilities to the max. I had twenty-four students in a six hundred square foot classroom with no window. This was not an ideal place for this student.

He did not last very long in our school. After a particularly trying morning, I kept him back in my room while the other students went to a specialist. His behaviors were bizarre at the very least. He climbed on top of a six-foot bookshelf that jutted out into the room and refused to come down. As I stood next to the bookcase, partly to provide a safe landing if he jumped and partly to use proximity to make him get down, I looked into his eyes. I will never forget the feeling as he blankly stared at me and spit full in my face. His eyes revealed nothing, a complete lack of conscience.

Within a month, this student had assaulted me by hurling snowballs at my face as hard as he could from a distance of less than six feet. At the time, I was restraining his violent younger brother who had attacked a vulnerable younger student. He then sucker punched me in the face, bloodying my nose and breaking my glasses.

In another incident, he took a large broken eight-foot branch and chased our female principal while threatening her. His younger brother exhibited many of the same behaviors. What I didn't know then was both brothers fit the profile of FASD. A meeting with their parents convinced me the boys did not have the structure for success in that family.

Another boy, a fifth grader, was continually in trouble. He would assault his teacher, assault other kids, was incredibly impulsive, but when he could contain himself, was kindhearted and talkative. He was very attached to his female teacher, but was so volatile she had to be very careful whenever she was with him.

One day, an urgent call came to me to assist with him. He was running through the school with a fire extinguisher, threatening everyone who got near him. He was swinging it like a chunk of wood, striking the walls and anything in his way.

This young boy did not have a chance in life. He was a heavily impacted FASD child who had no supervision or care at home. The only place he found hot food was at school. One day I went to his house to try to talk to an adult. The dirt yard was littered with refuse. The front door had a hole punched next to the doorknob, with a string hanging through the hole with which to pull to unlock the door. No one was home.

After I had been teaching at the school for a year, a nurse came to the school and presented on Fetal Alcohol Syndrome (FAS). I remember this day as the "Day of My Enlightenment." For the first time, I was able to put a name to what I was seeing on a daily, no…hourly basis. I watched and listened with complete amazement as the facts of FAS were laid out in front of all the staff of the school. Here was the root cause of all I was witnessing. The faces in the presentation mirrored the faces in my classroom. The behaviors brought on by fetal exposure to alcohol, as explained by the nurse, were the behaviors displayed by my students. The presenter's graphs of academic levels could have come from our California Achievement Tests. I did not need to know if the mother had self-reported drinking during her pregnancy. I saw the evidence first hand.

These students grabbed my heart. Even through the anger explosions, the physical assaults toward others and me and through the verbal outbursts of language directed at me, I was drawn to these needy students. I spent many hours and days outside my teaching responsibilities providing many different outdoor experiences for them. I served as assistant leader and within a year was the leader of the Boy Scout program, taking the boys on a four-day canoe trip on the first sixty-seven miles of the Mississippi. We spent four days on Lake Kabetogama, a beautiful lake on the edge of the Boundary Waters Canoe Area and a weekend hunting ducks on Lake Winnebegosh, one of the premier walleye fishing lakes in northern Minnesota. I taught Hunter Safety and took the boys to camp at the Many Point Boy Scout Camp. We spent a couple of weekends at a nearby rendezvous camp sleeping in old time huts and cabins. We stayed outdoors in below zero temperatures to get our "Zero Hero Award," making our outdoor shelters and keeping fires going throughout the nights. We cleaned the highway right-of-way and took a trip to a big campout in Oklahoma.

Each of these outings further underscored the level of difficulty our students were experiencing in social skills, reasoning, memory, and physical wellness. They loved being outdoors, doing environmental-based learning, making fires and cooking campfire meals. They thrived on kinetic activities that could hold their interest. They enjoyed having another significant adult in their lives, an adult who did not fail them. I grew to know these boys very well, experiencing their night terrors, their impulsive fight or flight responses, their tender moments with younger siblings or friends, their explosions of anger and frustration, and their unrelenting penchant for making the wrong decisions at the wrong time.

On one canoe trip, as I paddled up to the bridge where we were to stop for lunch, one of the boys was standing at the landing, ready to tell me something that I would have never believed could happen. His partner, a sixth grader with a history of academic and behavioral problems, had refused to stop along side the river to relieve himself. Instead, he dropped his shorts and defecated in the canoe, right in front of the disgusted paddling partner.

I was, on those occasions, as were the other participating adults, their "seeing eye brain", always there to remind them, to channel their thinking, to give their brain a nudge so it could rethink.

Unfortunately, not all the significant adults in their lives were providing good supervision. One evening, two of boys who had taken Hunter Safety were playing with a shotgun in one of the boys' home. One took the gun and pointed it at the legs of the other and pulled the trigger. The other boy lost his leg from the knee down. The mom was tending bar in the small town on the reservation and dad was drinking at the bar when the shooting happened.

Not everything was bad. I have nothing but respect for the teachers at the schools where I worked. They are committed and responsible. They understand the difficulties they deal with on a daily basis. Their hearts are in the right place and they grieve at the amount of damage the kids display and they keep coming back. I had many good experiences.

A friend introduced me to the libretto of *The Phantom of the Opera*. I brought it to school and let my sixth grade students hear the score. These kids from the reservation, schooled in gangster and hip-hop music, couldn't stop listening to the music. We began a reading unit, culminating in a visit to a theater in St. Paul, 250 miles away from the reservation, to see the real performance. I couldn't have been more proud of my students as they sat in the plush theater and knew every word of the score.

In my fifth year of teaching, I took a job as the first full time principal for the then new Mille Lac Band of Ojibwe Nay Ah Shing School. Here I saw more of the same behaviors, with an increasing gang influence taking advantage of the limited brain capacity of the FASD students. As the principal, I was seeing entire families impacted with FASD. I saw mothers who had borne six kids with several different fathers. Each of the children were heavily impacted by prenatal exposure to alcohol, with the younger children having much greater difficulties from FASD than the older ones. Some of the students were so impacted they were years behind their peers, both in academic ability, emotional maturity, and physical stature.

In my second year as principal, a family of three sisters enrolled in the school. Their former school sent records that indicated the three girls had not been attending school. We did not have any record of the fifth grade student attending any school after third grade.

Needless to say, their academic levels reflected their lack of attendance. The only thing we were certain they had learned was how to organize the girls in the middle school into a gang. Within weeks, the girls were banding together with the leaders being the three sisters. Not only were they threatening violence in the school, we were hearing they were acting out the violence in the community.

As staff, we intervened and were able to gain control of their actions. The girls' mother did not like the fact we had to discipline her daughters. One day she came into the building without checking in at the office. I intercepted her in the hallway and asked her to go back to the office so we could talk. Her response? She attacked me, kicking me in the groin, narrowing missing where she was aiming. She was modeling what her daughters were acting out.

One of our students was a large, slow, ungainly boy, who was unable to keep up with the curriculum. His mother was a heavy drinker with an volatile temper who had lost her job at our school when she was caught purchasing alcohol for underage students. This young man, who was emotionally several years younger than his chronological age, struggled with his weight, as well as reading and math. He would come to school with strange hairdos. He missed many days of school, choosing to stay home in bed. His mother would lie to cover for him. He had an explosive temper. One day, he attacked a teacher with classroom scissors. Fortunately, his choice of weapons linked with his slow movements, gave the teacher the chance to avoid his attack. He continued to go to our school under specific requirements. Knowing what he was capable of, we continually provided a safe environment for the adults working with him while still giving him every opportunity for success. We avoided putting him into situations that would trigger his outbursts.

The community was not talking about the overwhelming reality of FASD behaviors. When I met with an incoming new police chief and spoke to the number of adults and students who were brain damaged from FASD, I was chastised for using the phrase "brain damage." The leaders of the reservations said and did little, as their children and relatives were victims of FASD.

I was responsible for the educational programming, so I began to seriously research what was known as Fetal Alcohol Syndrome at the time to see how we, as a school, could provide the most optimal educational environment and experience. I felt like I was a lone voice when I talked about the issues, but I continued to develop and implement programs, with the support of my superintendent, that were specifically designed to give FASD children the best school experience possible.

I began to see a direct link between heavily impacted FAS kids and gangs. Mille Lacs was experiencing a staggering increase in gang activity and our school was a hotbed of recruitment. Two major gangs were establishing territories and the schools were included in their turf. We quickly began to realize our enrollment in the middle school and high school was more dependent on what gang the students belonged to rather than any other factor. One family ran one gang and another family made up the bulk of another gang, and both were linked to gangs in Minneapolis and St. Paul.

Our school was the school of choice for one of the gangs. Any member of the opposing gang who was forced to go to our school, by their parents or, because they had been expelled from the public school, met immediate threats of violence unless they left the school. We were constantly on guard for fights and retaliation. Most of our middle school and high school students were much more concerned with who they were aligned with than any reading or math lesson.

As our school spiraled downward trying to cope with the gang influence, I began to see a pattern. Our heavily impacted FASD kids were the enforcers of the gangs. They were the ones who would fight at the flash of a sign or at the command of their gang superiors. They were the ones who didn't think about the consequences of their actions. Our school was the turf of one of the gangs and a sixth grade student was the gang leader. I watched as high school seniors deferred to this sixth grade student. This was a new experience for me and I was determined to get the upper hand.

A family moved to a town about thirty miles away, trying to get as far away from the cities as possible, but still be able to attend our school. The mother enrolled her son and asked if we would accept the enrollment of a friend who was an eighteen year-old senior with a felony and a long gang history. He seemed polite and he met the school's tribal enrollment criteria. I was in for a ride with this young man.

Over the course of the next several months, I got to know him very well. He was polite and reserved, but there was an edge to him. Many evenings I took him home after basketball practice, a trip that added more than thirty miles to my evening commute. During these times, he opened up to me, telling me of his gang experiences involving violence and murder in the heart of Minneapolis and St. Paul. He wanted to get out of that life and had attached himself to this family as a way of garnering a supportive group of people to help him.

I saw him as one of the few students I had worked with who did not display the brain damage behaviors of FASD, but willfully chose the path he walked. Years later, he proved me right by becoming a hardworking licensed member of the construction trades and leading a fulfilling life. His painting on the wall of my office constantly reminds me of his struggle to successfully rid himself of the gangs.

Our young gang leader at the school was not happy we had this eighteen year-old at the school. Our newcomer was from the wrong gang and ignored our young gangster. The tension started to build. One afternoon, I stepped out of my office and saw the gang members circling our commons area, with the senior, all senses alert, ready to defend himself. They were moving as one, the gang members on one side and he on the other. Apparently an order had been given and the gang was making sure the order was carried out.

We were able to break the attention away from the lone gang member, but the damage had been done. He had been challenged and he was not going to back down. We had to have the St. Paul Police Department intervene and have him picked up on a probation violation. I clearly saw how the gang was impacting our school and how anyone who did not meet their expectations as a gang was subject to threats and violence.

I needed to isolate the leader. I brought him into my office. He came from a violent family whose mother was a gang member and a heavy drinker. He fit the profile of an FASD juvenile. His reading level was several grades lower than his chronological age. He was accomplished at getting what he wanted through either his fighting or his authority in the gang given to him by his very violent brothers, one who had been expelled from our school for tapping a bullet on a desk and telling a teacher it was for her, and two others who were gang chiefs in the state penitentiary.

Within minutes, he was crying, telling me he did not have a choice. If he left the gang, he would be sought out by the gang and either beaten within an inch of his life or killed. He believed that with everything in him. He could not see a way out of his life. In his gang life, he constantly worried who would beat him up, what his mother would do to him, or what store would she want him to rob. He told me the structure of the gang, who were the leaders in the community, what his role was and what he was told he needed to do. His role was to train the young fifth, sixth, and seventh graders into gang members. The detail was frightening.

As he spoke, I realized he was telling me the truth. His brothers had assigned him to be the "leader in training." He was not old enough to lead the reservation gang made up of older teens and adults, but he could train new gang members in his young gang. Within a few years, he would then be moved into the leadership on the 'rez,' as the reservation was known. He was to recruit students who would not have fear, who would fight when asked, and would follow the direction of the gang. In other words, he recruited the FASD kids, both male and female. Before they could be gang members, they would have to prove themselves.

To prove themselves, the gang had a very specific set of tests. To get to the first assignment, the recruit would have to be "beaten in" the gang. The gang members would surround and beat on the recruit for sixty seconds. A new member' first task after being "beaten in" was to attack and beat up a random person pointed out by the young gang leader or one of his inner circle of gang members. He described how they would walk around and point out someone for their recruit to attack. This person may or may not be from the reservation. He or she may be a visitor to the casino. After the recruit passed the first test by thoroughly beating up the victim, they would be given an assignment to attack and thoroughly beat up a member of the rival gang. Passing this test, the recruit would then be assigned to attack a specific member of the rival gang. If the rival gang member retreated to his or her house, the recruit was to break windows in the house until the gang recruit and his followers were let in. If this did not work, the recruit was to set fire to the house. If the recruit accomplished all the required missions, he or she would be eligible to become a member of the big gang.

I reported this information to the tribal police. Two weeks later, a house within two hundred yards of the school was set on fire after that identical sequence of events played out. This was no "wannabe gang." Our gang was for real, but the community and parents turned a blind eye. I don't know how many times I heard, "Not my kid!"

Drive-by shootings were happening with increasing regularity. Gang members from the Mille Lacs reservation would drive up to Leech Lake and do a drive by shooting and the Leech Lakers would retaliate. The violence seemed to escalate each year. October seemed to be the most violent month, as the darkness came earlier and it was still warm enough to be out and around. Grandparents told me of huddling in their houses on Friday and Saturday nights afraid to walk out to their car because of hearing shots up and down the streets. Yearly, kids would be airlifted to St. Cloud or Minneapolis with serious head injuries due to beatings with golf clubs, bats, and even a mailbox. A former student, heavily impacted with FASD, killed his cousin in a drunken fight. A girl in our school was so severely beaten into a gang, she could not come to school for a month due to the condition of her face. Girls could be found doing a web search for their boyfriends on the state penitentiary website. And this was in a school of less than 150 middle school and high school students. Now, several of those faces adorn the pages of the state penitentiary website. Our young gang leader is now earning his advanced training in gang leadership as an inmate of the state.

I saw a clear link between the violent actions of the gang and the FASD kids in our school. The gang members, with very few exceptions, were the kids who exhibited behaviors consistent with heavy prenatal exposure to alcohol. The environmental factors of their lives clearly exacerbated their propensity to be involved in wrongdoing.

The Brain Damage Revealed

What I was experiencing, but didn't fully understand, was physical deformities are not the only evidence of damage caused by prenatal exposure to alcohol. I was looking for the physical evidence of facial indicators and linking what I saw to the accompanying exhibition of brain damage. A psychologist friend urged me to attend a workshop put on by Dr. Ann Streissguth, one of the preeminent researchers in FASD. She is a Professor Emeritus in the Department of Psychiatry and Behavioral Sciences, at the University of Washington School of Medicine. As a licensed clinical psychologist with a specialty in behavioral teratology, she has studied the effects of prenatal exposure to alcohol for over 30 years. Two hours of listening to Dr. Anne Streissguth further opened my eyes and confirmed that what I was seeing in the classrooms and hallways of the schools was irrefutably Fetal Alcohol Spectrum Disorder.

Her entire presentation was focused on the brain damage of fetal alcohol exposure without any accompanying physical indicators. She presented animal research studies exposing the extent of brain damage suffered by fetally exposed animals that did not have the revealing facial features of Fetal Alcohol Syndrome. Her presentation was powerful and life changing for me. Now I could see clearly. The greater share of the damage was hidden from view, hiding behind the social mores of the society, seemingly acting in collaboration with the makers of alcohol, damaging without showing how and where, keeping the populace in the dark, growing within the population like a hidden virus.

This powerful little lady described a scientific study of rats and how prenatal exposure to their brains impacted their ability to control their impulses. A study, replicated to ensure consistent results, revealed significant brain damage at levels of exposure that do not result in facial deformities, a condition called Fetal Alcohol Effects (FAE).

Rats are impulsively afraid of the light. When exposed to light, they seek darkness. In this experiment, the mother of the rat was given alcohol while pregnant, enough to damage the brain, but not enough to cause physical deformities. The FAE rat was then placed in a cage that had a portion covered to provide darkness. In that darkened area, a shocking device was placed.

A normal rat, when the light was turned on, would go into the darkness, get shocked, and return to the lighted area. It would stay in the lighted area, shaking, but resolute, controlling its impulse to go into the darkness because it did not want to get shocked.

The FAE rat that looked exactly like the normal rat, would go into the darkness, get shocked, rush out into the light, impulsively go back into the darkness, get shocked, rush out into the light and continue to do the same until the researcher stopped the experiment.

As she spoke, I could see the same damage with the kids from my schools. They would be disciplined for a behavior and impulsively repeat the same behaviors time and time again. They could not link their action to the consequence of their action. The discipline, while rightly administered, did not have an effect on changing their behaviors.

Streissguth continued. Researchers knew they could inject enough alcohol into eggs to damage the brain of the chick, but not have any effect on the physical appearance of the chick. These chicks were then placed in a holding area in a pen that had an open side door and a plexiglass window overlooking a bowl of chicken feed with a couple of stooge chicks eating away. Among the damaged FAE chicks were some normal chicks. The FAE looked identical to the normal chicks. With a couple of pecks on the window, the normal chicks moved around and found the open side door, moving quickly to the bowl. The FAE chicks pecked away at the plexiglass, wanting to get to the feed, but were unable to think beyond their fixation. After some time, the researchers guided the FAE chicks to the open door.

The next day, the experiment was replicated. The normal chicks pecked a couple of times and moved to the open doors and hurried to the feed. The FAE chicks had not learned. They pecked and pecked at the window. After some time the researcher guided them to the open door.

This continued daily. After five days, some of the chicks learned. Some never did. These chicks did not display any physical signs of prenatal exposure to alcohol, only behavioral signs of the brain damage of prenatal exposure to alcohol. Again, this experiment was replicated with the same results.

I sat in my seat thinking about how this study revealed so much about the children I had worked with. So many times had I taught a lesson, only to have to re-teach and re-teach for many of the kids. We had purchased powerful software for our students just for that reason. A computer does not get angry with a child if the same concept has to be presented time and time again.

She was not done. This time, Dr. Streissguth presented a research study on mother mice who were FAE. The experiment studied the ability of a brain damaged mother mouse to protect and care for the infant mice. A nest was built on one end of the cage. The infants were placed at the other end of the cage. The researcher wanted to see if the FAE mother had the instincts and ability to bring the infants back to the nest.

Undamaged mother mice were given the same task. When timed, the normal and FAE mothers, who looked identical, raced to the end of the cage and brought the first struggling, squealing baby back to the nest in the same or close to the same time. That was when everything changed. The normal mouse continued to diligently race back and forth, with a singular focus on the safety of her babies, bringing all of them into the protection of the nest. The FAE mother mouse, on the other hand, raced to the other end of the nest, picked up the second baby, stopped midway between the nest and the squealing babies on the other end, dropped the one in her mouth, raced back, picked up another one, raced forward, tripped over the one in the middle, stopped, befuddled with noise on each side of her, being unable to focus due to all the commotion. Her brain, damaged from prenatal exposure to alcohol, could not tune out the sensory inputs of her babies squealing from both sides of the pen. The quickest an FAE mother mouse got her babies back to the nest was eighteen times longer than a normal mouse. Some of the FAE mothers finally stopped, with babies spread out from one end to the other.

I sat rooted in my chair. I was daily seeing mothers who were struggling with the most mundane of motherly tasks. Many of the students in my schools were living with grandparents because the mothers and dads had discarded their children to the grandparents' care. Now, what I was seeing made sense. This epidemic of brain damage did not go away when the child reached adulthood. It was just exhibited in a different way and our society was being overwhelmed by the impact of prenatally exposed children who became adults and who then had more prenatally exposed children, most of whom needed social services.

FASD and Schools

As I struggled with the challenges of teaching FASD children in the reservation tribal schools, I saw similar behaviors and attempts at remediation with students in public schools. I was seeing that this "condition" was virtually unrecognized off the reservations. Because of my experience on the reservations, I had been given the opportunity to witness this first hand, to be able to "see clearly", to be able to look at my family, my home town and my state to comprehend how all of us are being impacted by children and adults who were fetally exposed to alcohol.

In the late 1990's, an article from the National Indian School Board Association (NISBA) was sent to each of the 184 Bureau of Indian Affairs (BIA) funded schools. This paper placed the blame for low reading scores of Native American students directly on the dominant culture and the lack of books of interest to Native American children. I was not surprised with this point of view because I had been hearing this for years, but there was no Gold Standard research to support the contention. Once again, this paper had completely missed the elephant in the middle of the room. Nowhere in the white paper was any mention of the level of impact fetal exposure to alcohol was having in the schools. I wrote a letter to the Executive Director of NISBA to that effect, but was ignored. I clearly saw the victimization of the Native American people, but now understood there was a deeper root cause for the learning problems I was witnessing that was unrelated to the victimization.

Victimization of the children by the dominant culture is a favorite crutch in the tribal education system. One day, a neighboring school's students came to Nay Ah Shing School to experience the Ojibwe culture beading classes being held by one of my favorite elders. She was quite excited after the students from the other school left. When I had the opportunity to speak with her, she could not stop talking about how those "white kids" learned so much easier than the tribal kids in the school. That did not fit into the politically correct notion that all that is needed to have the tribal students learn at the same rate as the rest of the nation is to provide culturally relevant materials. When comparing our tribal students and the neighboring school's white students, our native children struggled to learn using culturally relevant beading, in the same way we experienced with their reading and math. The same root cause for the difficulty of learning existed for both experiences.

Three years of consulting across Indian country after my tenure on the Mille Lacs Reservation further opened my eyes to the extent of FASD. A job opened up in Fort Hall, Idaho. I was hired and spent two years as the Superintendent of the Shoshone Bannock School District #537. This junior and senior high school was the epicenter of alcohol abuse and Fetal Alcohol Spectrum Disorder for southeast Idaho. While I was at the school, six young people, either students or children of employees, were killed in alcohol related accidents. In fact, the day I left the school to move back to Minnesota, I received a call while I was driving across Montana, telling me a girl who had graduated two weeks before had been killed the previous night in an alcohol related auto accident.

The academic and behavioral characteristics of the majority of the students in the school were indicative of fetal exposure to alcohol. A local teacher, a tribal member, came to my office one day after school and, in the midst of our conversation, said that at least 70% of the students in her class were FASD. My observations of the students during my two years in the school support her claim. In this school, as in my other schools, a high percentage of students struggled in reading and math and had behavioral problems.

Many times I would see a small, heavily impacted FASD fifteen–year-old running down the halls of the high school. He was a friendly kid, likeable, but very frustrating if you did not understand his brain damage. He could not remember to bring a pencil to class. He was late more times than not. He teased kids for attention and was bullied and pushed as a result. He kept coming back for more.

This undersized kid was bullied and teased because of his size and race. He came to our school because we understood how to work with students with FASD, or at least most of the staff did. One day, a new teacher to our school, with 40 years experience in public schools, came to me boiling over with anger and frustration. She demanded that this student should not come to her class anymore. He had once again come to class without a pencil and she had belittled him for forgetting. He blew up, and she continued to berate him by saying things such as, "What do you think I am, a bookstore?" and "Why don't you act your age?"

Of course he was not acting his age because he had the emotional age of a ten year old. His emotional development was not delayed; it was arrested. He would never act his chronological age. He would never be able to remember everything we normally would expect a person his age to remember. But, some of the adults around him expected and demanded he act his age. They disparaged him when he didn't. He used the only survival skill he knew how to use, anger. Through that anger, he would be removed from the trying situation that triggered him. Once he had triggered, exploded, and calmed down, we could talk about what happened, with the unfortunate reality it would happen again, and again, and again.

This is one example of many I could make where the actions of the professionals working with FASD children made the situation worse. The shaming and blaming language by professionals who do not understand brain damage drive prenatally exposed adolescents to the debilitating secondary disabilities of FASD, such as depression, violence, disrupted school experiences, and trouble with the law.

Because of students such as him, I initiated and implemented a program designed for FASD children called the Intensive Services Program (ISP). This program was so successful several non-native FASD students from the public schools surrounding the reservation enrolled in this Bureau funded school specifically to be served in our ISP classroom.

The day the disturbed shooter, Seung-Hui Cho, killed 32 college students at Virginia Tech, I testified at a Federal Tribal Consultation in Billings, Montana, on the diametrically opposed Tribally Controlled School Act and No Child Left Behind (NCLB). At this consultation, I told the Assistant Secretary of Education and the Bureau of Indian Education Director the one single factor impacting student achievement I have experienced in the tribal schools was the high incidence of Fetal Alcohol Spectrum Disorder and the resulting low achievement in reading and math. Their disdain for my testimony was palatable and shown not only in their verbal response, but in their non-verbal expressions. There was no room in their mind for any deviation from the "All children will be proficient" stance. They would not consider the evidence or even the possibility that children had brain damage that would preclude them from meeting the expectations of the NCLB. That is what I call the "Arrogance of Authority." Here were people in positions so removed from children or so impressed with their authority that they can not see the truth or even consider the possibility that someone has a clearer vision than they of what is occurring.

It was during my tenure in Idaho that I acted on my sense of urgency to tell people what I had experienced and could now identify. I wrote an Insight Article for the *Idaho State Journal* titled, "A Deadly Link." The piece was published April 15, 2007, one day before the Virginia Tech campus shooting. At that very time, Pocatello, Idaho was immersed in the trial of two sixteen year-old boys who had done the unspeakable; murdered a female classmate to experience the thrill of killing. Did anyone ask if they were prenatally exposed to alcohol? No. Did at least one of them fit the profile? Yes.

By writing this article, I had stepped out of the school building and into the public with the intent to enlighten as many people as I could to this epidemic.

Throughout my career, this sense of urgency continued to move me to learn as much as I could about fetal exposure to alcohol. More and more I realized we, as a society, have no idea as to the real impact mothers drinking during pregnancies has on our schools, communities, and entire society.

CHAPTER Three
The Challenge: We Can't See the Damage

We Think They Think the Way We Think They Should Think

While serving as the principal at Nay Ah Shing School in central Minnesota, I sat on the advisory board for the local newspaper. I found myself questioning time and time again why the paper was not looking into the impact of fetal exposure to alcohol in the community. The relative disregard for my questions and concerns by the publisher and editor was an indication to me that we, as a society, did not know or were unwilling to find out, the impact prenatal exposure to alcohol was having in our communities. It was fine to look to the reservations and complain about how alcohol was decimating the reservation and to write stories about how people were helping the women on the reservation, but it was unthinkable to consider our community was being affected with the same epidemic.

I emailed news reporters locally, statewide, and nationwide when I would read articles that stated causes for people's actions without looking at the possibility of fetal exposure to alcohol. Only a few reporters responded and none had asked or even considered the possibility of a connection.

One evening I watched a news magazine report on a research project with death row inmates. All of the death row inmates had minimal electrical activity in the frontal lobes of the brain. I remember pounding my fists on the table in frustration when there was absolutely no mention of prenatal exposure to alcohol mentioned as a possible root cause for the limited functions of the frontal lobes of the brain. Not only were the reporters ignorant of the impact of prenatal exposure, the researchers did not have a clue.

In most everyone's mind, for an individual to have a Fetal Alcohol Syndrome, the person must have the "look" (and even then, few recognize the syndrome). The "look" is that of the classic, heavily impacted Fetal Alcohol Syndrome (FAS) child. Those children, affected by the resulting brain damage, are obviously expected to be lower functioning and then receive services through the schools and other human services (without officially recognizing that the child is a victim of the syndrome). FAS is only the tip of the iceberg. By far, the greater share of brain damaged individuals do not have any facial characteristics. Most of the time, FASD remains undiagnosed and the behaviors are classified under some other label. I have found very few professionals who understand or have taken the time to learn that the physical syndrome features of FASD are only a small part of the entire spectrum. The victims of prenatal exposure to alcohol who have none of the classic syndrome features are the kids who are at great risk because we think they should behave and think normally.

After I had my eyes opened to the brain damage that can be revealed through both academic and social behaviors without seeing physical deformities, I began to see evidence of FASD in murders, violent acts, in stories of foster children, in national stories of child abuse, sexual abuse, and parents abusing children. I began to build a matrix in my mind to evaluate every story, every incident, and every struggling student I worked with. I studied abstracts of research to refine the matrix in my mind. What I began to see has brought me to the point of writing this book.

The research is clear and unequivocal. Alcohol is a powerful teratogen. Lead is a powerful teratogen. Alcohol and lead are the only two teratogens a woman could ingest that kill the brain cells of the fetus. Women drink alcohol, not lead. A teratogen is defined as an agent "capable of causing serious harm to the fetus. Because alcohol causes central nervous system damage, it is also classified as a neurobehavioral teratogen" (Alcohol, A Potent Teratogen, Medscape.com). This cannot be said often enough; alcohol is a teratogen and as such is much more damaging to the brain than meth, cocaine, or crack.

Bluntly said, a woman's drinking during pregnancy damages the brain. Damaged brains do not function like normal brains. Damaged brains cause people to do things a normal person would not do.

A recent *Minneapolis Star Tribune* headline screamed, "Police Know Who, But Do Not Know Why." We are asking questions without knowing how to look for the root cause. Whenever I saw something abnormal, deviant, or out of the ordinary, I would apply the matrix. I began to look for "red flags," details surrounding events or people's lives that gave me indications the mother of the perpetrator exposed the child to alcohol during the pregnancy. I looked for persistent behavioral indicators, both academic and social, that fit the matrix. I was disturbed with what I began to see. I ask you, no, I beg you to prove me wrong, because if I am right, our society has no clue as to how we have been impacted by brains damaged through fetal exposure to alcohol.

The brain of the fetus is damaged many ways. The frontal, temporal, parietal, and occipital lobes, the hippocampus, the hypothalamus, the corpus collosum, the cerebellum, amygdala, and the basil ganglia all suffer varying amounts of permanent injury that exhibit in behaviors. Individual brain cells die, neurons are damaged and cells migrate to the wrong locations. Research continues to confirm ethanol in the alcohol is the culprit. **Longitudinal studies confirm the brain damage is irreversible.**

In each of the incidents reported in the news, I also look for the "red flags" shown through physical deformities. Pictures and physical descriptions of the subject can reveal FASD in several ways, although many of the facial features tend to be less prevalent as the child moves into adulthood. Birth defects in the form of physical deformities include small stature, small head, slack muscles, lack of the defined structure between the nose and lip called the philtrum, thin upper lip, epicanthal folds between the eye and nose causing the appearance of almond shaped eyes and a greater distance between the eyes than normal, other facial anomalies, heart problems, kidney problems, hair growth on the back of the neck, genital deformities, eye problems, shortened and/or bent fingers, hip deformities, pigeon or concave chest, cleft palate, spinal dimple, and/or hernias.

Adopted children, unfortunately, are at a very high risk of having been prenatally exposed to alcohol. American families, to avoid adopting a "crack baby" from the United States, many times have adopted undetected brain damaged FASD children from Romania, Bulgaria, and other middle European countries. The unsuspecting adoptive parents are then overwhelmed with the litany of problems as a result of the biological mother's drinking that led to brain damage. Simply put, who are the mothers who abandon their babies or put their babies up for adoption? The vast majority are young mothers who don't want or can't take care of their babies. These unborn children are at great risk of being the victims of binge drinking by the young mothers.

A longtime friend invited me to a cup of coffee at his country place. The hours went by as we reminisced about our many adventures over the years. Eventually, I brought the subject around to my book and asked if he could reflect on some of the incidents that I write about in this book. Somewhere in the conversation I mentioned the fact that one of the school shooters had a birth defect known to be a result of prenatal exposure to alcohol - a concave chest. A peculiar look came over his face. I waited, knowing he wanted to say something.

Up to this time, I think he felt FASD was someone else's problem. The look on his face was revealing. This man was someone who was never at a loss for words. This was one time he thought carefully before speaking.

His parents had adopted three of his cousins, all siblings from a German aunt who was a heavy drinker. He told me how the mother had abandoned the children. The connection was made when he heard about the concave chest. His adopted brother had a concave chest. My friend was deep in thought as he spoke. Furthermore, he told me his adopted brother had a heart attack at the age of twenty-five, another indicator of the birth defects of prenatal exposure to alcohol.

Research and the Brain

Studies show women drink during their pregnancies at unbelievable rates. Binge drinking is linked to unplanned pregnancies and binge drinking is especially damaging to the child. Studies show drinking one half of a drink a day can lower the child's language skills. Drs. Joanne L. Gusella and P.A. Fried found even light drinking (average one-quarter ounce of absolute alcohol daily) could have adverse affects on the child's verbal language and comprehension skills. (*Neurobehavioral Toxicology and Teratology*, Vol. 6:13-17, 1984)

A 2001 study revealed that an adverse behavior effect can result from an average of one drink per week and children with any prenatal alcohol exposure were 3.2 times as likely to have delinquent behavior scores in the clinical range compared with non-exposed children. (*Pediatrics*. Vol. 108 No. 2 August 2001, p. e34)

Studies show a link between fetal alcohol exposure and lower dopamine, the chemical linked to Attention Deficit Hyperactivity Disorder (ADHD) and Attention Deficit Disorder (ADD). Further studies show a link to Autism (http://pubs.niaaa.nih.gov/publications/arh25-3/199-203.htm)

A study entitled, "Causal Inferences Regarding Prenatal Alcohol Exposure and Childhood Externalizing Problems," (*Archives of Genderal Psychiatry,* vol. 64, no. 11, Nov. 2007), found that conduct problems in children increased for each additional day of the week on average that the mother drank while pregnant.

This research involved 4,912 mothers and 8,621 of their children and ruled out many other explanations for the conduct problems, in part, because the investigation included multiple children per mother. This permitted researchers to look at siblings who were prenatally exposed to alcohol at different rates because their mothers had varying rates of drinking during different pregnancies. The study found that children more frequently exposed to alcohol during pregnancy had more conduct problems than their siblings who were exposed to less alcohol prenatally. Conduct problems identified in the report included such behaviors as intentionally breaking things, bullying, cheating and lying. The researchers also concluded that children whose mothers drank alcohol during pregnancy also had more attention and impulsivity problems.

A 2008 study by researchers at the National Institute of Environmental Health Sciences (NIEHS), part of the National Institutes of Health, found that pregnant women who binge drink early in their pregnancy increase the likelihood that their babies will be born with oral clefts. The researchers found that women who consumed an average of five or more drinks per sitting were more than twice as likely than non-drinkers to have an infant with either of the two major infant oral clefts: cleft lip with or without cleft palate, or cleft palate alone. This study only looked at the physical deformity and did not examine the co-existing brain damage. (American Journal of Epidemiology /Advance Access published July 30, 2008.)

When and how much alcohol consumed is the major determining factor as to how much damage, where the damage is, and how debilitating the damage will be. This condition has had many different names: Fetal Alcohol Syndrome (FAS) used when physical deformities are evident; Fetal Alcohol Effects (FAE) used when the physical deformities are not evident, but the brain damage is evident; Alcohol Related Neurological Disorder (ARND), Alcohol Related Birth Defects (ARBD) to name a few. Sometimes I think we should call them Alcohol Babies because a similar phrase worked to get the message out about for Meth Babies and Crack Babies.

The term Fetal Alcohol Spectrum Disorder (FASD) was coined to encompass the entire spectrum of brain damage from the minimal loss of potential to the death of the fetus. As indicated by a spectrum, not all areas of the brain may be damaged; some may be spared significant damage. Damage may be so small, brain scans may not reveal the damage, but the damage is real and exhibited through behaviors of the child or adult.

An FASD victim may have an IQ of 140, but not be able to maximize their IQ due to other parts of the brain being damaged. On the other hand, prenatal exposure to alcohol is recognized as the single greatest cause for mental retardation and the only totally preventable cause.

According to Dr. Anne Streissguth, (*Final Report from Research on Secondary Disabilities* presented to the FAS Conference in Seattle in September of 1996) the academic abilities of individuals with FASD are below their IQ level, and their living skills, communication skills and adaptive behavior levels are even further below IQ levels. Because the damage is directly linked to the time and amount of exposure, victims of FASD show none, some, or all, of the spectrum of behaviors.

Specific areas of the brain are linked to both academic and social behaviors. The large complex frontal lobes of the brain are vital for speech, planning, problem solving, social behavior, self-awareness, and impulse control. Many of the exhibitions of behaviors of FASD children are connected to damage of the frontal lobes. These behaviors are exhibited through impulsivity, lack of understanding of personal space, limited ability to problem solve, and poor personal hygiene, to name a few. The executive functions of the frontal lobes will be explored further in this chapter, as this part of the brain is particularly hard hit when prenatally exposed to alcohol.

The portion of the frontal lobes known as the occipital lobes are vital to visually recognizing objects and understanding what written words mean. Many FASD children struggle with written comprehension. In my many years of experience, I have witnessed a high number of students hitting a plateau in reading when they reach the third grade, the grade level when comprehension becomes the mainstay of the reading programs.

The temporal lobes are vital for memory and emotion, as well as hearing and understanding language and sounds. Memory is a very difficult process for many FASD children. Limited emotional control is a behavioral indicator that can't hide in the back of the classroom like poor comprehension can. This brain damage, when linked with damage to the hypothalamus, is displayed by temper tantrums, inability to control emotions, anger, instant friendship with anyone (making them very vulnerable to sexual abuse), illogical love/hate relationships, and depression leading to suicidal tendencies. As with all brain damage, this is irreparable. Our jails are filled with people who have brain damage exhibited by the lack of emotional control,

33

resulting in the death or harm to others.

The parietal lobes are the collector of messages from the other parts of the brain. Connections are made and interpretation of sensations and messages happen in the healthy parietal lobes. Touch, temperature, sounds, visual information of the surroundings are inputs to the parietal lobes. This important part of the brain also aids in understand shapes, sizes, and directions. Many kids forget their coats, mittens, boots, etc., in cold weather and do not seem one bit concerned about the effects of the cold.

The corpus collosum is the major super highway between the right and left hemispheres of the brain. Damage in the corpus collosum interferes with the ability to pass information from the left hemisphere of the brain to the right hemisphere. The left hemisphere plays a large part in language, verbal memory, reading, writing, and arithmetic skills. The right hemisphere plays a large part in interpreting what we see and touch, non-verbal memory, music, and emotions. When damaged, the corpus collosum superhighway is many times downgraded into a county road, or in the most severe cases, a cow path. I have recorded a significant amount of data over the years that show a plateau in the fifth through seventh grades, when the arithmetic changes from skills and memory to the abstract of algebra. The damaged corpus collosum limits the ability for the math skills developed in the left brain to be interpreted as algebra by the right brain. The damaged brain remains locked in a concrete thinking mode.

Damage to the hippocampus, located in the medial temporal lobes, effects long term 'declarative" memory and learning. Declarative memory is made up of facts, figures, and names you have learned over the years. The importance of the hippocampus is illustrated in the medical journals when a patient, only known as H.M. had most of his medial temporal lobes removed in an effort to quell his epilepsy. Since his surgery in 1953, he has made no new memories. He can remember his childhood and up to his surgery and has a working memory, but if you leave the room for a moment and come back in he will not remember you or what you were talking about. Without his hippocampus, he has lost all memory retention function.

FASD clearly impacts the ability of children to remember facts and figures. The hippocampus has been identified as one of the brain components most impacted by prenatal exposure to alcohol. In my experience, math is particularly difficult for many FASD children and adults. The damage is very evident when the hippocampus is not fully functional.

The amygdala is to emotions as the hippocampus is to memory. This segment of the brain controls the body's reaction to fear. It connects a learned sensory stimulus to an appropriate response. Damage to this part of the brain can be seen in a child who has no fear of strangers, or when an older child or adult does not have the protective fear of going into strange places, walking about in the dark, or, as in the case of the gangs, being the enforcers of the gang. This lack of fear is a common behavior exhibited by heavily impacted FASD individuals.

Damage to the hypothalamus limits control of appetite, emotions, and temperature and pain sensations. Many FASD kids have a high pain tolerance. Cerebellum damage wreaks havoc with coordination and movement as well as behavior and memory.

The basal ganglia, a group of structures around the thalamus, are important for voluntary movement and voluntary thought, a funnel, so to speak, where thought gathers. People with severe damage to the basal ganglia, such as Parkinson's Disease, lose the ability to control movements and lose the body's innate ability to use sensory input to voluntarily move or fluidly think. For instance, a person with severe basal ganglia damage would not be able to interpret the sensory input when they place their foot partially on a step, thinking the foot is fully on the step.

Damaged basal ganglia would exhibit the behavior of only focusing on one behavior without the ability to do two or more at once. For example, to cut a steak, one needs to saw the knife back and forth while putting downward pressure on the knife. One with severe damage to the basal ganglia will only move the knife back and forth because the brain will not be able to integrate the modes of thought into one voluntary action. With this damage, the brain literally cannot focus on more than one item or issue at a time. Thinking slows down and becomes "thick", because of the inability to deal with two or three issues at a time. In the more severe cases, the limited single item focus drains the brain of any ability to work toward goals. This characteristic also limits the ability of the brain to link behaviors to consequences. Many violent actions by brain damaged individuals are a result of the "thick" thinking, the fixed focus on a solution that is illogical and unrealistic, the inability of the brain under stress to move from the singular thought, not allowing the brain to think about the consequences of that thought.

In 1848, Phineas Gage, a young likable man of exemplary character with a good future ahead of him, became the subject of the most unlikely study of brain damage as it relates to human behavior. He was an employee of the Rutland and Burlington Railroad and was working with explosives while blasting rocks for a new stretch on the railroad. As he was tamping down the blasting powder for a dynamite charge, he inadvertently caused a spark. The dynamite exploded. This explosion drove the one inch thick, three foot long, thirteen pound tamping rod shooting up through his cheek, through his brain, and out the top of his skull. He dropped to the ground, convulsing, then stood up and started talking to his co-workers.

His shaken co-workers loaded him on an oxcart and took him to the nearest hotel. Doctor John Harlow dressed his wounds. Gage remained alert and talking throughout, even when Dr. Harlow stuck his index fingers into each hole until his fingertips touched. As he did this, the young man asked when he could return to work.

Within two months, Phineas Gage recovered, although he lost one eye. He could walk, talk, and demonstrated a normal awareness of his surroundings, but the former Phineas was much different from the new Phineas. Instead of the dependable, likeable, moral man he had been before the accident, he was now an anti-social, foulmouthed, immoral, ill-mannered liar given to fantastic schemes he never completed. Dr. Harlow observed, "The equilibrium between his intellectual faculties and animal propensities seems to have been destroyed." He lived for eleven years after his injury and his behaviors did not change or improve.

In the case of Phineas Gage, the change in his behavior was completely understandable. The evidence of brain damage was immediately observable due to the outward signs of facial damage and the loss of his eye. The resulting behaviors were attributed to the accident. Recent studies by neurobiologists Hanna and Antonio Damasio of the University of Iowa of his skull and the trajectory of the tamping rod using computer enhanced imaging revealed damage to the lower frontal lobes, called the ventromedial region. The other regions of his frontal lobes necessary for language and motor functions were untouched.

The descriptions of Phineas Gage's transformation can be extrapolated to much of the brain damage suffered in the womb by so many of the prenatally exposed children. Unfortunately, these victims of frontal lobe brain damage are branded. Descriptions such as ill-mannered, immoral, delinquent, insolent, rude, disrespectful, antisocial, social misfits, are 'wired wrong", a "bad seed" are common. Most are considered willfully disobedient because they look just like any other kid and you can't see the damage to the frontal lobes and other regions of the brain. We expect them to learn or change, but many times, they do not have the capability to change in the same manner as Phineas Gage couldn't change. Some can only manage their behavior in situations where there is little or no stress. When the stress of depression, anger, frustration, sexual hormones, adrenaline, or other common occurrences overwhelm the damaged brain, the capability to manage their behavior diminishes dramatically. The same goes when alcohol and drugs are introduced to the damaged brain.

The executive functions of the prefrontal cortex are highly likely to be disrupted or affected by the teratogenic exposure to alcohol. These executive functions are a result of the frontal lobes controlling inhibitions, sexual urges, problem solving, verbal expression, planning, working memory, motor control, time perception, self-monitoring, judgment, motivation, and, as exhibited with Phineas Gage, provides a moral compass. When the frontal lobes are damaged by fetal exposure to alcohol, the resulting behaviors can range from a minimal impact to severe behavioral characteristics. One victim might display difficulty with his working memory or difficulty with the abstract concepts of time and money, but not be aware this is caused by prenatal exposure to alcohol. Another might not be able to control impulses, continually having to refocus on the task at hand because every movement, every sound, every bright color in the room impulsively draws attention from the task at hand.

Prefrontal cortex damage, when linked to other damage of the brain, exhibits in a behavior that is frustrating for parents, educators, and the courts. The inability to control an impulse linked to the inability to understand the consequence of an action, puts the damaged brain into situations where the individual is punished for an impulsive behavior without learning to stop the behavior. This double whammy of misunderstood actions is played out countless times in schools and in juvenile courts.

Students who are disciplined one day for an offence are back in the office the next day for repeating the same offence. Stronger and stronger punitive actions are followed by the same behaviors, seemingly without having any effect. How many times have you heard of the offender being incarcerated in the juvenile system and when released, re-offends? When I explained this brain damage characteristic to a police detective several years ago, he said this was the first time someone gave him an explanation that made sense regarding the behaviors that he was experiencing on the street.

The Exhibition of Brain Damage

Recently, I conducted a study of prisoners in the Crow Wing County Jail, located in Brainerd, Minnesota. This regional facility receives prisoners from surrounding counties and as far away as Texas. Twenty-five percent of the inmates responded to the research survey. The Assistant Program Coordinator felt this was a representative sampling. Of these inmates, ninety-four percent had mothers who drank alcohol. Five of the responding inmates volunteered to be interviewed. Of that five, all fit the profile of FASD. All had mothers who drank alcohol, all had siblings who were exposed, and three had children who were exposed. One reported eight siblings, children, fiancé, and stepchildren who were fetally exposed to alcohol. The inmates who were interviewed came from both high-income families and low-income families. Prenatal exposure to alcohol damage happens to all incomes and ethnicities. Our prisons and jails are full of people who have frontal lobe damage and other brain damage that inhibits their ability to make good judgments, their ability to link an action to a consequence, their ability of self-control, and their ability to control their sexual impulses.

Attention Deficit Disorder (ADD) and Attention Deficit Hyperactivity Disorder (ADHD) are two of the main characteristics exhibited by frontal lobe damage where impulse control resides. In the vast majority of cases, psychologists, special education specialists, medical doctors, and psychiatrists do not recognize the causal relationship between prenatal exposure to alcohol and ADD/ADHD. If you wonder why so many of our children are being medicated, please start to ask the question: Did the child's mother, through consumption of alcohol, expose the child to any alcohol during fetal development?

After a board meeting of a local non-profit organization recently, four board members and I visited about our futures. As I explained my plan of writing a book and of speaking about my experiences with FASD, the conversation turned serious. One of the board members, a friendly, gregarious thespian, whose life was in shambles, spoke of her mother's drinking and how the descriptions of impulsivity and other characteristics of FASD were descriptions of her. Another woman, a retired accountant, asked if there were any reasons other than prenatal exposure to alcohol that may be the cause for her daughter being overly impulsive, as neither she nor her husband were impulsive. I could not give her an answer. As we left the meeting, she pulled me aside and asked if I drank. When I said I was a light social drinker, she said she was the same. She left trying to remember how much she had drunk during her pregnancies. She did not have any knowledge of the damage brought on by her drinking at the time she was pregnant. Now she was aware any level of drinking had put her children at risk. Now she had some information to provide some answers.

The inability to follow a sequence of directions is a major characteristic of FASD brain damage. In a classroom, the typical direction from a teacher may include a sequence of several specific sequential details, such as; "Go to your desk, get out your Social Studies book, turn to page 34, and begin reading at the third paragraph." A child with FASD will be able to follow the first direction, but will have great difficulty remembering the second of the sequence of directions, and forget the rest of the directions. But she/he will be expected to do what the rest of the class has been told to do, and will be chastised, and most likely shamed and blamed, if he or she does not follow directions.

Recently, I had a parent meeting to talk about a particular student who exhibited all the physical and behavioral characteristics of FASD. The meeting went well. His father was the only parent at the meeting. He agreed with all the observations the teacher and I had regarding the academic levels and behaviors of the child. I asked the teacher if this student had difficulty following a sequence of directions. She gave examples of times when he would follow the first direction, and then stop, with a questioning look on his face, trying to remember what he was expected to do.

His father, a veteran, whose epicanthal folds around the eyes looked suspiciously like someone with FASD, said he had the same academic and behavioral problems as his son. Specifically, the father had a problem remembering directions. He described how, when he was in the military, he would have to write down standard operating procedures and sequences of directions as his superiors would give them, so he could remember them.

As the meeting came to a close and the other professionals had left the room, I asked him if his boy had been prenatally exposed to alcohol. As we both had come from the same northern Minnesota area when we were young, he laughed and said everyone was drinking where he came from. He said his wife was a heavy drinker and his mother was a heavy drinker. He had no idea what Fetal Alcohol Spectrum Disorder was and was grateful for any information I could give him. After seeing the information on FASD and knowing the level of drinking in his family, he recognized FASD was most likely the issue both he and his son were struggling with.

Understanding the damage to the executive functions of the brain and to the emotional control in the temporal lobes is crucial to understanding the FASD individual. Brain damaged students with a roller-coaster of uncontrollable emotions can be dangerous to themselves and others, played out in the form of suicidal or angry aggressive actions. I have witnessed both in the extreme. This lack of emotional control, when linked to another damaged executive function, such as judgment, the inability to weigh the pros and cons when making decisions, can be dangerous to the child and others. These conditions, coupled with the inability to switch modes, to generalize, to link the behavior to the consequence, and the limited ability to control emotions can be explosive or move the child to a self-destructive depression.

Many times, the damage combines to limit the person's ability to have what we call a conscience. The FASD person takes actions without thinking about the consequences, and then, when the consequences of the action are presented to the FASD person, he or she can't understand how it is linked to what he or she did. This is a common characteristic of FASD. Knowing this trait is critical in understanding the lack of a conscience exhibited by so many kids and adults.

A man who was born of alcoholic parents recalled a day, when he, still a kid, went into the barn where a bunch of wild cats were running about. He told the story of how he wanted to pet one of the cats. He caught the cat, which promptly started scratching and clawing. He continued to grip the cat, so focused on petting the cat, he was unaware of what he was doing to the cat. The cat continued to fight until it died. This man remembered all he could think about was wanting to pet the cat. He was fixated on his desire to pet the cat and the result was an arm all scratched up and a dead cat. His disappointment was not that the cat was dead; it was that he did not get to pet the cat.

This is a dangerous characteristic of brain damage. Simply put, some FASD brains fixate, whether it is on shoelaces, a pencil, or a person. This behavior gets more frightening when the fixation focuses on a person, and the FASD child is experiencing the hormone rushes of puberty. There is ample evidence of boys thinking a particular girl is their girlfriend, when in reality the girl has only been helpful and friendly. The fixation moves to harassment and violence. The example of the boy wanting to pet the cat, and holding it until he killed it, is an example of fixation, on the wanting to pet the cat without any thought of the consequences of that act, or what he had to go through to get what he wanted. I believe this is the root cause of many murders of women by their spouses or boyfriends. In many cases, genuine remorse follows harmful fixated actions. The perpetrator can't believe or understand why he did what he did.

This fixation, when linked with alcohol, can be serious. In news reports detailing a court case from Canada, comes an example of the illogical fixation caused by raging hormones, alcohol, and brain damage. A mother and daughter were loading groceries into their van. A fifteen-year-old boy, identified in court as having FAS, climbed into the van. He had been drinking. His brain was fixated on sex. The mother told him to get out of the van, but he sat without saying anything. Suddenly, in plain site of others in the parking lot, he attacked the mother, mauling her chest and groin in a clumsy sexual assault. People came to her rescue upon hearing her screams. This boy, who had been mired in the foster system in Canada, is now a criminal, one of the countless FASD individuals who sit in prisons everywhere.

Many times the behaviors resulting from the brain damage are baffling. One day the brain may seem to remember, the next day, be unable to. One day the brain seems to cope with a situation, the next day the brain does not have the capability to do so.

Many times, the survival skills of the FASD child mask the real levels of damage. An FASD child may have good verbal skills with little or no comprehension. The verbal skills may give a teacher the belief this child can work at grade level, but in reality, the child uses verbal skills to get out of work that is beyond his capability, thus giving a false impression of his ability. I can't tell you how many times I have heard teachers say the student is smart and can do the work, but, when I analyze the writing and reading skills of the student, the teacher has been fooled into thinking the student had the skills and ability. What the teachers did not have was the right tools to assess the student's abilities.

Another child may use avoidance through behaviors, giving the teacher the belief the child can do the work, but does not want to. This confusing exhibition of behaviors typically puts the child into the category of willful disobedience and is a huge source of frustration to teachers and parents.

A clear "red flag" for prenatal exposure to alcohol is impulsive behaviors that appear to be uncontrolled by the child. While there are other biological causes, when impulsive behaviors are linked to other prenatal exposure indicators, the probability of prenatal exposure is much stronger.

One day I was observing a little girl trying to finish her assignment. The mother confirmed her daughter was fetally exposed to alcohol. No physical characteristic, other than small stature, was immediately evident. I watched as her attention continually was taken away from what she was assigned to do. She wanted to do the work, but was unable to concentrate. Again and again she tried to refocus, but something in the gaily decorated room would draw her attention away from the task at hand. I could see she really tried to do her work. I could see she was getting frustrated because she could not focus. I came away from that observation with the understanding she had every intention of doing what she was assigned to do, but her brain would not let her concentrate on the task.

This type of impulsive behavior completely traps the child in a world of constantly changing impulses. Animal research studies clearly link alcohol exposure to brain damage exhibited by limited to no impulse control.

I have witnessed many students who would explode with foul and hateful language when he or she didn't get his or her way with a teacher or another student. These students knew they would be removed from the room, but they couldn't control the impulse. Within minutes, they would be remorseful and ready to continue in the classroom, classic examples of brains damaged from FASD.

One evening, I stood in the line at the local Wal-Mart in southeast Idaho, completing my purchase. Two security guards in civilian clothes rushed past with radios in hand. They positioned themselves on both sides of the exit, waiting for an unseen person to appear. I nonchalantly walked past, expecting to exit without causing a stir. Once outside, I glanced back into the store. There, stuffing clothes behind the pop machine was one of our junior high students. He straightened up, looked me full in the face, and then continued to frantically shove his armload of stolen merchandise out of sight.

I now knew why the guards were waiting. They would act when the merchandise left the store. Sure enough, a car pulled up, honked, and he grabbed his loot, tore out of the store, ran right in front of me, giving me an insolent glance, not caring I had witnessed his law-breaking and, seemingly gleeful, he had pulled it off. His glee turned to shock when the security guards exploded out the door and grabbed him and the stolen goods.

He was the first violent student my new assistant principal had to deal with. Within the first two weeks of school, his impulsive violent behavior pattern became evident. In a friendly game of basketball, another student grabbed a rebound away from him. His immediate reaction was a sucker punch to the face of the unsuspecting student. Adults intervened and he was escorted to the office. I pulled the assistant principal aside and told him any policy we had would not be a deterrent on a student with his disability. We could suspend, suspend, and suspend again and not make an impact because he displayed all the physical and behavioral characteristics of FASD. I told him this student would react impulsively with violence, and without a conscience, but he would not be able to connect a consequence to any behavior. The assistant principal did not believe me. Within months, he was a believer. This student continued to behave in the same violent manner, assaulting students and staff, verbally and physically. No punitive action had any effect.

He was one of the few students I have worked with who had such significant brain damage, along with non-supportive environmental factors, that not one of the strategies we could employ worked. The adults he lived with denied his involvement in these behaviors, compounding the problem. His brain thrived on the emotion and adrenaline of violent and lawless actions, especially when he could get support from his uncles. Eventually, he quit coming to school, even though we ran a separate bus route to fit his guardian's schedule.

This young juvenile was a survivor in a difficult environment. He was quick to fight, quick to anger, quick to explode in a verbal fury of profanity laced insults. He did not seem to care if his victim was an adult or someone younger. If anyone got in his way, he reacted. He would lie without batting an eye. He delighted in making up stories that shocked people. One day he instigated an investigation of animal cruelty when he came to school telling people he had gotten angry at his horse after being kicked. His story took a sinister turn when he boasted he had taken a gun from his grandmother's house and shot the horse in the belly. Hours later, we found out he was telling a lie.

This student exhibited the entire range of a heavy level of brain damage and was already a criminal by the time he was 12 years old, with literally no hope of living a life outside the confines of the local tribal jail or the state prison as he moved into adult life. His story is similar to that of many of the other students I worked with, both on the reservations and off.

In one school, a sixth grade student was sent to me because of his argumentative behaviors. This youngster was someone I had taken under my wing, as he and his teacher would come to loggerheads over assignments and teacher directions. He is a bright, athletic, friendly, and clean cut kid; someone you would never think would be struggling with issues. I observed his behaviors from the standpoint of brain damage, as I knew he was taking medication for ADHD.

He had a quick smile and seemed to be doing well in school. But the clues, the "red flags", were there. He perseverated, a behavior exhibited by the tendency to continue or repeat an act or activity after the cessation of the original stimulus. He could not stop when he started to focus on an argument, like a dog with a bone, shaking it, chewing on it, and worrying it until something else takes his attention. His teacher and I worked with him, putting him on a contract so he could analyze his behavior in an attempt to make changes in his behaviors. For the most part, he was successful. Occasionally, an explosion happened. Books and papers flew, and then he would crash, falling into a pool of depression. Usually this was a byproduct of a change of medication or a confrontation with his stepfather, a man with little patience for this youngster's problems.

One day, he and his teacher did not see eye to eye on an assignment. He started his perseverative behavior, not letting the teacher get the last word. He ended up in my office.

These were the times I looked to find a strategy to change his behavior without being punitive. His actions were a function of his disability, even if he did not have a special education determination. I showed him the paperwork I needed to accomplish to do my job, as an example of what he could expect when he entered the workforce. Eventually, I gave him some of my professional writings to edit as an assignment. I told him he was the first one to put eyes on this work other than me.

He took his assignment seriously. The next day, he came to my office to talk about what he was reading. I will always remember him sitting at my table and saying, "This is why my brother is like he is. He has the same thing I have." When I gently probed, he said when his younger brother was born, his mother had a boyfriend who was a heavy drinker. I told him that would not have resulted in FASD. "Yes, I know," he said, "But my mom's boyfriend had a big influence on my mother." His younger brother was already taking Ritalin and struggled at school. This youngster's insight into his mother's drinking patterns led me to believe he was prenatally exposed to alcohol also, an observation that was supported by his behaviors and prescribed medication.

He is one of the prenatally exposed kids who would never be thought of as FASD because he did not fit the profile of an insolent, academically challenged physically deformed misfit. In a way, his predicament was as great or greater. The adults around him do not see any physical indicators of brain damage. He is one of the 70% of FASD victims without any physical characteristics who has been and will be looked on as a willfully disobedient individual and punished as such, a factor that could very well drive him to depression and violence.

Unfortunately, death is one of the outcomes of prenatal exposure to alcohol. At one of the schools, a small student with all the indicators of prenatal exposure, including confirmation his mother drank, excitedly informed everyone of his new sister's arrival. Two weeks later, his excitement turned to despair when his baby sister was taken to the emergency room where she struggled to stay alive. Within two weeks of her birth, she died.

He brought the obituary to school as a way to work through his grief. My heart sank when I saw a picture of this little girl. Her face, so innocent and sweet, could not hide the clues of heavy prenatal exposure to alcohol. Her opportunity to live was taken away one binge at a time.

Brain damage from prenatal exposure to alcohol is not a respecter of ethnic, religious, or geographic boundaries. Our judicial system is full of men and women who have this damage. Our schools are overwhelmed with the challenges brought to their doors by children with this little understood brain damage. Our education system is reeling with the expectations of success that will never be met for students with this brain damage. Adult FASD males are swamping the judicial system. Adult FASD females are flooding the social services system with entire families of FASD children, and unwanted or uncared for brain-damaged babies. Teenage FASD girls are having unwanted and unplanned pregnancies, exposing their children at alarming rates. Teenage boys are committing violent acts that are clogging the juvenile systems and putting many of them in adult courts due to the nature of the violence. Babies put up for adoption are overwhelmingly FASD. As is said in the FAS community, the girls get knocked up, the boys get locked up.

Our country's FASD population is growing at an exponential rate. In my experience, it was common to see four, five, and six children in the same family with two, three, and four or more different fathers. These children were prenatally exposed to alcohol and struggling immensely in school. Within fifteen years, the children were having families of their own and prenatally exposing them to alcohol, many times abandoning them to grandmothers and the foster system. The vicious cycle continues, adding more FASD children every generation.

The only way to start to stem the tide is to understand the depth of the problem. We need to start asking the question every time a violent or deviant act takes place, every time a student is assigned a Special Education Individual Education Plan, every time a mother gives birth, every time a child is medicated for behavioral reasons, every time a criminal is tried in court, every time an inmate is incarcerated, every time a person becomes a client in the social system. Only then will we know how much a mother exposing her fetus to alcohol impacts us all.

CHAPTER Four
It Can Happen to Anyone

While my experiences in the epicenters of prenatal exposure to alcohol are unique and brought me an understanding few have of the devastation of FASD, the rest of my life could be categorized as normal. That is, until I started analyzing behaviors within my family I had been witnessing throughout my life. I believe anyone who reads this book needs only to look within his or her extended family to understand how much prenatal exposure to alcohol is impacting our society. Some of my normal family had become abnormal over generations because of generational prenatal exposure to alcohol. I tell you this at the risk of alienating some very dear people, but I can't keep quiet. I apologize if I offend some of my family. Please know I do this because of the urgency of the message.

Any mention of drinking alcohol to my mother would bring a quick chastisement and a response from the scriptures. Because of the fear of disappointing my parents, I did not venture into the world of drinking alcohol until I was married. Even then, I was cautious, not wanting to lose control of myself. I can remember the first alcoholic drink I ever had, a Golden Cadillac, enjoyed after a fine dinner with my wife at a local restaurant. I was a twenty year-old college student when I met my future wife, a beautiful brown-eyed girl who was willing to ride on my motorcycle. Had she known my nickname was "Crazy Crowe", she might not have gotten on the motorcycle the first time. I was on my own and ready for some adventure, something that had eluded me while living with my parents.

A whirlwind romance resulted in our engagement and subsequent marriage a year after we met. My wife was an experienced drinker, growing up in a wonderful friendly family of German heritage, where beer, wine, and hard liquor were vital components of every family event. Her small North Dakota hometown celebrated Christmas with Tom & Jerrys set out for anyone at local businesses, and the local bars were the central social locations during the long cold winters. Family events were punctuated with frequent trips to the basement to get beer from the refrigerator. Comparisons of taste and texture of beer and wine were commonplace. I had married into a different culture, a culture of alcohol, and I did not know how much that culture would impact me in my future professional life.

Within three years, we started a family. My wife conscientiously refrained from ingesting any aspirin, over the counter medicine, alcohol, or any other potentially harmful food during her three pregnancies, with two exceptions. She allowed herself one beer with each of the first two pregnancies, exposing two of our three children to a small amount of alcohol.

My wife's sisters and brothers continued to drink during their childbearing years and fetally exposed most of their children to alcohol at varying rates, just as they had been exposed by their mother. The pattern, started well before anyone had much understanding of the dangers of prenatal exposure, continued on, with grandchildren being exposed prenatally. My mother-in-law, a truly wonderful person, sat with me one day and told me what was done could not be changed. In fact, her doctor had told her to drink alcohol.

My daughter, after being preached to about the risk of drinking during a pregnancy and after bringing me to school to talk to her Family Living Skills class about FASD, exposed her children to alcohol when she was pregnant. A niece, an alcohol baby herself,

50

abandoned her newborn twins to her parents, who raised the two children as their own.

While I clearly saw the exposure, I did not yet see the resulting evidence of brain damage. Only after I began developing programs in schools for FASD children did I look into my family and clearly see how we were impacted for a lifetime by our actions as parents. Of all the members of this family, over two thirds were fetally exposed to alcohol. Of these, one shows facial and physical characteristics of FASD, four exhibit social and academic behaviors of FASD, two were prescribed Ritalin, and several more could be described as having a loss of potential due to exposure to alcohol.

My wife's family is a good family, a well-respected family in the community. They are practicing Lutherans, not missing a Sunday. I enjoy being with them. I love them and cherish my time with them. It pains me to see what alcohol has done that cannot be undone. I am so grateful all the children are being brought up in structured families, which will provide the optimum environment for success.

When I was young, I remember my family reunions on my mother's old family homestead, with most of my forty plus cousins gathering at my uncle's farm, across the road from Grandma's house. Horses, ball playing, and horseshoes were the activities of the day.

Growing up on that far north farm surrounded by the balsam and tamarack swamps, my grandparents raised their eleven children as hardworking men and women. The siblings did not have access to alcohol in their younger years. They were miles from the nearest town and nearest church. Their lives were wrapped up in scratching out a living in the woods and fields of northern Minnesota.

Only after my uncles left the farm and the strong supervision of their stern mother, did alcohol start having an effect. Stints in the army gave these farm boys a taste of the world. Two of the brothers married women who were known to drink alcohol and some of resulting offspring were decidedly different than the other cousins in the family. It wasn't until recently that I realized why.

One uncle and aunt had six kids and a litany of issues. Both my uncle and aunt worked at the lakeside bar. One of the prenatally exposed boys was born with a concave chest, which was somewhat of a wonder for our young eyes. Another uncle and aunt were constantly in the local bars, a fact not known to our family at the time but confirmed by a police officer as I was researching for this book. Their oldest child displays physical and academic characteristics of FASD. Only when my eyes were fully opened to FASD was I able to understand what I had been seeing throughout my life. Only then was I able to ascertain the root cause of the difference between the cousins. It was not entirely genetic. The drinking of the mothers as well as the academic, behavioral, and physical indicators were there to support the reality of prenatal exposure to alcohol.

Conversely, when my father's side of the family gathered in Kentucky, I did not see any of the characteristics related to FASD. My grandfather was proud of the fact that several of his grandchildren entered the ministry of their church. I am not trying to make this a religious issue, only stating a fact. Some churches look the other way when members are imbibing. Others condemn drinking like my grandfather's church did. One of my dad's sisters married a man who drank alcohol, but she did not drink. The other siblings married spouses who did not drink. In looking at my cousins, I do not see any of the academic and social behavior indicators that I have seen in the rest of my extended family.

Revealing the facts of my family has been a soul searching, wrenching decision, but, if I am to be brutally honest with others, I need to be painfully honest with myself. I apologize to any family member who may be offended with my observations, but please forgive me and please look at the facts. FASD is everywhere, and affects so many more people than anyone can imagine.

Almost daily, as I continue to step up on my soapbox, people relate their private experiences with me, experiences they usually do not speak about because so few people understand. Most think they are the only ones who are dealing with this problem. Many have no idea they have been struggling with a child with brain damage caused by prenatal exposure to alcohol. Time and time again, I have watched as mothers, especially mothers of adopted children, begin to understand what has been creating so much anxiety and guilt in their lives.

My willingness to talk about my experiences has provided others the opportunity to talk about theirs. At a weekly service club meeting, a highly regarded businessman visiting our club energetically engaged me in a conversation about FASD after I had brought up the subject. He seemed relieved to talk to someone who understood what he and his family were going though. His story did not surprise me. His was one I had heard several times from countless parents.

He and his wife adopted a son. Their dream of having a loving relationship dissolved into years of seeking help for the multitude of problems they were experiencing. Finally, after having to take their son to a professional over three hours away, they found the answer, an answer that gave them a name, but not a prescription to heal the symptoms. Their son was permanently brain damaged by the pre-natal exposure to alcohol by the birth mother. Within my small circle, this was one of many examples of the hidden epidemic in our world.

A young Christian couple adopted two baby girls, totally unaware that one of their daughters had been exposed to alcohol before birth. Led by the adoption agency into believing that all was well, they expected to raise two normal, healthy sweet daughters. It wasn't until one girl, in her teenage years acted totally out of character from who her parents had known her to be. At that point her parents began to grasp that something was very wrong. All the unusual behaviors in their daughter growing up were soon going to begin to make sense. They found out about FASD for the first time from a local agency whose outreach was to families in crisis. This family then had their daughter tested for this disorder. The verdict was in. FASD explained their daughter's strong impulses, her outbursts of anger, her dilated eyes that caused her to have regular headaches, her overly concrete thinking as a teenager, and her inability to process life normally. After opening her adoption case, they found files that showed the birthmother answered every question on the form about her life, except for one. She did not answer the question asking about her drinking during pregnancy.

The adoption agency did not require an answer to that question. Their family could have been spared operating in the dark all those years concerning the unusual behaviors in their daughter. They could have helped her sooner, if they had known what was going on inside of her.

A business owner came to me asking for advice. He had adopted two children, birthed by his sister who had been drinking during her pregnancies. His adopted son was tantrumming and his behaviors were escalating. He was asking what to do, as he knew I worked with children with similar brain damage. He and his wife were struggling with their guilt about their parenting skills also. All I could really tell them was to keep his son's life highly structured, as that is the strategy that will provide the most success. Also, if they were to seek professional help, make sure the practitioner had a good understanding of FASD.

A pastor of a small church in a northern Minnesota town adopted three children. He and his wife were wonderful parents. As the three children grew up in the church congregation, the parenting and the children's actions did not seem to be congruent. The parents harbored much guilt about what their children were doing. No punishment worked. His children were getting into trouble in school and at church. All three were having difficulties. His oldest daughter ran away at sixteen and one of the boys was more vulgar and offensive than the other. This pastor and his wife were raising three children who were highly impacted FASD children, but the uninformed members of the congregation simply regarded the children as willful juvenile delinquents.

I spoke to my daughter's Living Skills class when she was in ninth grade. After my presentation I had time and asked for questions. The girls were very interested and inquisitive. Then, out of the blue, one of the girls said, "That's what's wrong with my brother!" She went on to explain that her mother and father divorced when her mother was pregnant with her brother. She could remember her mother going on an extended drinking binge. The result was a brother who had behavioral problems, who would tantrum and who had academic difficulties.

A local banker adopted three girls, offspring from a local woman who was known as a heavy drinker. He and his wife experienced varying levels of behaviors from the three, with the middle child exhibiting the greatest behavioral challenges.

The list goes on and on. After speaking to a group of superintendents and principals, the gentleman who coordinated the event told me of his adopted brother, who was highly impacted with FASD. Another superintendent inquired about me speaking in his community, as he had adopted two children, one of them most likely FASD impacted.

After working with me for two years while I was a superintendent in Idaho, a colleague came back from a nephew's funeral with opened eyes. He had originally thought I was crazy when I talked about FASD. Two years working with the population of students on the Shoshone Bannock Reservation had opened his eyes to what had happened in his own family. On that Monday morning, when he returned, the shock of losing a young nephew was deepened by his realization that not only was the nephew who had died a prenatally exposed person who had struggled through life, but that there were others in his family with the same profile. Both of his sisters drank alcohol throughout their pregnancies. One of his sisters drank a strong concoction of vodka and other hard liquor prescribed by her doctor. His nephews had exhibiting throughout their lives some of the same characteristics he was seeing in the students in our school.

Each of these parents, siblings, or relatives of FASD children could write a chapter in my book. Each has different, yet similar, experiences of ignorant professionals, inaccurate diagnoses, and children who defy the common academic and behavioral patterns of normal children. Each of these parents could tell many stories of other adults who believe the behaviors of their FASD children were the result of poor parenting.

I tell you about my family and the other acquaintances and colleagues to emphasize the depth of the problem. Research is clear on the amount of exposure our children are experiencing. **This is not only an Indian reservation problem. This is a national problem.** The Center for Disease Control analyzed data from the 2002 Behavioral Risk Factor Surveillance System Survey (BRFSS). The results were an indictment of our society. Women of childbearing years are drinking at a staggering rate. At the time of the survey, over 50% of women 18-44 years old reported drinking alcohol within the past month. Over 54% of women who indicated they did not use birth control and might become pregnant reported alcohol use within the preceding 30 days, with over 12% of the same women reported binge drinking (five drinks at one sitting) in the past 30 days. Up to 21% of all women reported binge drinking.

Further national studies substantiate this data. In a study

published in Pediatrics (Pediatrics, 2003;111:1136-1141), nearly half of all pregnancies in the United States are unintended. This study of over 72,000 women shows binge drinking is associated with the risk of a woman having an undesired pregnancy. This study also found women who were binge drinkers before pregnancy were more likely to be white, unmarried, smoke, and be exposed to violence. They were also more likely to drink alcohol and smoke during pregnancy.

In 2002, the Minnesota Department of Health commissioned a study entitled *Taking a Closer Look; Drinking During Pregnancy in Minnesota*. The results should have made headlines. As could be expected, our government and news media have been very successful making sure we know about illicit drugs. In Minnesota, 61% of women think cocaine is the ingestible drug most harmful to their fetus. In fact, the majority of Minnesota adults think crack or cocaine is worse for the baby than alcohol. Almost everyone, 97% of adults, know something happens when a pregnant mother drinks. A surprising 43% cannot specify what would happen if an expectant mother drinks. Women with a history of drinking are the most likely to think drinking is not risky to the fetus. What the media has not reported with any consistency is the fact that alcohol kills the brain cells of the fetus and, as such, is a much greater teratogen than cocaine, crack, or meth.

When asked if their doctor informed them of the dangers of drinking during a pregnancy:

- 33% of mothers said their doctor did not mention alcohol at all during the pregnancy
- 20% were advised to drink lightly or in moderation.
- **Only 37% were advised to not drink any alcohol during the pregnancy.**

In the national studies cited previously, over 50% of women reported drinking. In the Minnesota Department of Health report 62% of all women of childbearing age are "current drinkers." Over 22% of women in Minnesota self reported binge drinking at least once a month (5 drinks in one setting), statistically comparable with the reported 21% nationally. A disturbing 25% of Minnesota women reported drinking at least once during their pregnancy with 12% self reporting consuming 5 or more drinks a month during their pregnancy. **At least 5% self report binge drinking during their pregnancy.**

The Minnesota study identified women who were **at risk** for drinking during pregnancy. The risk factors were:

- Single
- College educated (most likely to drink)
- Working in high level white collar jobs
- Younger (college aged) or older (35-45 years old)
- Affluent – over $50,000 income
- Living in the Metro

The study found that high school educated women drink less often, but drink higher quantities. Binge Drinkers factors include:

- being single
- young (under 30)
- less educated, less affluent smokers, use illicit drugs
- employed in blue collar setting with male dominated occupations where a large portion of the workers are heavy alcohol consumers

Since 1985 the number of Minnesota women who self-reported binge drinking has fluctuated between 8% and 13%. Binge drinking is much more common than chronic drinking, which has remained at about 5%.

These figures become even more distressing when honesty of reporting is studied. In a study done by the University of Boston of Public Health, **71% of women who drank during their pregnancy did not tell the truth when asked if they had drunk any alcohol in the past month**. This disturbing statistic was revealed by testing for markers in their urine samples. Another study using the meconium (the material found in the intestine of a newborn that is normally evacuated within 6 hours after birth) revealed between 18% and 24% of new mothers had consumed alcohol during the last 20 weeks of their pregnancy. This method of identifying alcohol exposure does not reveal any exposure during the critical first 16 weeks of the pregnancy, and more significant, during the first 6 weeks or more when the expectant mother may have no idea she is pregnant. A woman may quit immediately upon finding out she is pregnant and still bear a child with Fetal Alcohol Spectrum Disorder due to the alcohol she consumed before she knew she was pregnant.

Research consistently finds over 50% of women of child bearing years report drinking alcohol during their childbearing years. A woman may not know she is pregnant for up to two months or more. Over 50% of pregnancies are unplanned. This combination of facts reveals that more than 25% of fetuses are exposed to alcohol in the critical first four to six weeks, anywhere from a minimal exposure up to and including binge and chronic drinking.

The evidence of denial and refusal to change behaviors for the good of the fetus can be seen in this series of postings to a current website (http://babyrazzi.com/baby/2008/02/02/pregnant-women-choosing-to-drink-alcohol-in-moderation/#comment-174770). This site was a forum to discuss an ABC television report in which two mothers made different choices about drinking alcohol during their pregnancies.

I am 6 months pregnant and have had a few glasses of wine here and there. My baby boy is perfect. Perfect face, perfect organs, perfect brain and heart. He's kicking day and night, and this has been a wonderful, easy pregnancy. You people just love to make judgments.

The dead give-away that the alcohol issue is a moral issue and not a scientific one, is the language of the doctors themselves. They say that drinking is wrong, but if you drank before you knew you were pregnant, don't worry about it. So it's only wrong if you knew? Every woman should use her common sense. Don't get drunk, but 1 or 2 glasses is ok.

Hate me. I drank 1-2 times a week with my last pregnancy. Americans are scared sh...less to do anything including eating tuna fish when they are pregnant. Pregnancy is not an illness. If it's not good for you, it's not good for the baby. Everything in moderation.

Post from England

I'm in the UK where the attitude towards alcohol in pregnancy is different. I've never been pregnant in the US, although I am American by birth, but I've heard of pregnant women not being served coffee in Starbuck's because it has caffeine. Is that true?

I was far too nauseous to drink in the first trimester with any of my children, but I did have the odd pint or glass of wine after that and no harm done. With my first I craved a pina colada for WEEKS before I finally had one at about 36 weeks and it tasted heavenly. No one batted an eyelid, either. Old wifeys even recommended shandies as a source of iron.

There is a major stigma in the U.S. about drinking even very sparingly while pregnant. Drinking hard liquor or abusing alcohol while pregnant is unthinkable, but a few drinks of wine or beer during the pregnancy will not hurt your baby! I imagine that eating highly processed foods is probably way worse for your child! I would never advocate drinking, because I know that some people do not have self-control to have a small amount, but I do not think it is wrong to do so. Even my doctor said that it's okay if you are responsible about it.

My doctor said it was fine. In fact, she lived in Europe while pregnant, and drank regularly. It's the ABUSE of alcohol that causes problems.

Does it really matter? Who cares if u drink, all this talk about it harming the baby is a load of bulls***!

I have a 4 yr old son, I drank throughout my pregnancy (not all the time but the odd glass) and my son was perfectly healthy! So yes it is a load of bull!
People worry too much these days!

All what I'm saying is people overreact when it comes to drinking whilst pregnant, a pregnant woman can't tell anyone she's had a drink without being crucified.

This series of posts show the selfish or ignorant actions of mothers who drink for their pleasure without regard to what is happening to their child. The final post was the one I entered:

I am an educator who has worked for 18 years on reservations where over 80% of the children were victims of FASD, Fetal Alcohol Spectrum Disorders. You have been talking about FAS, where physical deformities are evident. That is only the tip of the iceberg. You are fooling yourself if you think you can drink and have a perfect baby. Maybe the baby looks perfect, but you cannot see the brain damage. I now work in a public school and the brain damage from FASD is very prevalent, as evidenced by the number of children in Special Education. Alcohol is a powerful teratogen, much more devastating than meth, cocaine, or crack. The ethanol in the alcohol interacts with the potassium in the fetus brain cells and kills brain cells. It interferes with the transfer of brain cells to their specific locations in the brain. It kills neurons. With every drink, you are taking potential away from your child.

Drinking at a low level, or at any level, for that matter, is like Russian Roulette, like holding a pistol, loaded with one brain damaging round to the baby's brain and pulling the trigger. One beer drank by the mother has the comparative impact of three or more beers for the fetus. A mother would never think of doing something like that, but the chance of taking away her baby's potential, even taking her baby's life, lies in the mother's decision to drink or not to drink alcohol. Every time she takes a drink, whether it is a beer, a glass of wine or a shot of liquor, the alcohol enters the baby's bloodstream and the loaded cylinder turns. Maybe the first baby does not exhibit brain damage behaviors, but be assured, the loaded chamber is there for the next child if she continues to drink while pregnant. The daily nightcap, one wild night, one binge with friends and the round is fired. What's been done cannot be undone and the gun is reloaded with more rounds for that child and the next because the pattern is established.

I recently met a mother who denied she had exposed her child to alcohol during her pregnancy. I gently told her I had worked for years with children who exhibited similar behaviors as her child. I asked her if she would look at some of the information I could provide her regarding FASD children. She eagerly accepted the materials, and then seemed to want to talk.

As I listened, she told me she had been doing drugs and drinking heavily before she knew she was pregnant. She said that as soon as she found out she was pregnant, she stopped both the drugs and alcohol. I accepted her admission. From what I observed with her actions and my observations of her child, I was not fully convinced however that she had stopped when she found out she was pregnant. After a lengthy visit, she seemed grateful somebody understood her child.

This information opened a door for her to take her child through. The mother had the courage to bring this information into the Individual Education Plan (IEP) meeting for her child. She asked for this information to be added to the IEP and had her child assessed. This is one of countless cases of the mother exposing her child before knowing she was pregnant.

The paperwork came across my desk for a new student. In the paperwork, a brief sentence fragment stated the student's mother drank alcohol during the pregnancy without linking this fact to the behaviors identified in the documents.

The student's father and father's girlfriend, accompanied by a social worker, came to the entrance meeting, bringing a folder stuffed with reports from doctors, psychologists, neurologists, teachers, and social workers. As the preliminary introductions and discussion ensued, I scanned the stack of reports. The father explained how his child had physical birth defects and a litany of behavioral problems in the current school, how one school worked for his child and the other didn't and how his child needed discipline rather than sympathy.

When an opening in the conversation allowed me, I asked the father about the biological mother's drinking habits. He described how she was a heavy drinker and tried to kill the fetus by punching herself in the stomach. That provided the opportunity for me to talk to him about the root cause of the birth defects, about the child's difficulties in school and home, and what we needed to do to meet the child's needs. I had his undivided attention. After about 30 minutes, he turned to his girlfriend and timidly apologized that he had tried to make her drink while she was pregnant with her new baby, which she refused to do. He said he had many of the same problems his child had and his own mother was a heavy drinker. In fact, his family had asked his girlfriend how it came to be that her new baby was so perfect. Now he knew; she had done something no other mother in his family had done in his lifetime, she had not drunk any alcohol when pregnant.

The next day, I learned he had told the school social worker he learned more from me in one hour than he had from any of his visits with his child's psychiatrist, psychologists, doctors, or neurologist. That is an indictment against the medical community and something that did not surprise me at all.

My family is not unique. My school is not unique. These students I have told you about are not unique. The parents of the students are not unique. The stories I have told you are not unique to Minnesota. They are only being revealed because they are under the scrutiny of someone with knowledge of FASD.

Many families have experienced what I have experienced, but do not know they have unwittingly taken potential from their children. Please open your eyes. Please, please, please do everything within your power to stop anyone within your circle of influence from drinking during a pregnancy. Give these babies every chance for success. The research clearly shows fetal exposure to alcohol is nationwide, is basically unknown and misunderstood, and is, for the most part, being ignored by the educational, human services and medical professions.

CHAPTER Five
Not in My Town! Eighteen Months from Hell

The hidden epidemic of prenatal exposure to alcohol is having a significant impact in every community. The brain damage is revealed through the actions of the individuals, but rarely does anyone realize the cause. News reporters write about the actions, lawyers argue about the cause of the actions, juries decide the outcome, brain damaged individuals serve the time, and taxpayers pay the cost.

One of the most visited small cities in Minnesota serves as an example of the hidden epidemic. Brainerd, the playground for the Twin Cities area, is the gateway to the spectacular lakes of Central Minnesota. Behind the hustle and bustle of this growing community of cities and towns, the specter of prenatal exposure to alcohol hides, ignored because of the community's lack of knowledge, much like any other community in the nation. Over a span of eighteen months, seven murders were committed. No one knew of the root cause or even knew how to look for it behind each of these tragic events.

December 24, 2001, dawned over this beautiful Minnesota lake community with children awaking in anticipation of the excitement of presents and the message of Christmas. Snow lay softly on the evergreen trees and the lakes lay dormant under the thick sheets of ice. Everyone was getting ready for the visit from that jolly old man of the north.

Angie and Ted Bieganek had a visitor with an entirely different intent during the night. Their early Christmas present was a bullet to the head, seemingly from an intruder who broke down the front door, killing them with brutal efficiency while they slept in their bed.

On Christmas Eve morning, Beiganek's grandson, Joshua DeRosier, drove up to their nice country rambler on Barbeau Road in his new pick-up. His grandmother, Angie, had helped Josh buy his pick-up by cashing in a trust fund to pay off his older pick-up, which he then used to trade in on his new truck. That Christmas Eve morning, Josh called 911 from his grandmother's driveway and reported something was wrong at his grandmother's house.

Within minutes of his 911 call, law enforcement officials arrived to take control of the scene. The front door was smashed in off its hinges, with glass strewn across the front room, but the interior of the house did not resemble a burglary crime scene. The Christmas tree stood undisturbed with presents tucked under the green boughs, ready for the family Christmas party they were to host that evening. Nothing else was disturbed. In the master bedroom, the two victims lay under the covers in their sleeping clothes, face down in the bed with fatal wounds to the head.

Investigators quickly narrowed their focus to one person, Joshua DeRosier. DeRosier had a history of disrupted school experiences and had not completed his high school course work at the alternative learning center. He had been in trouble with the law and, according to testimony, was on probation and could not have a gun for nine years. His parents were out of the picture and he had periodically lived with his grandmother and step-grandfather. He had many angry confrontations with step-grandfather Ted Bieganek. The Bieganeks had provided a room for him, but Ted Bieganek had recently given Angie an ultimatum that either Joshua left the house or he would. Angie had refused to continue to help Joshua with his high truck payments. DeRosier knew Angie had taken out credit life insurance policy on his truck payments and he told his friends the truck would be paid off if she died. Another friend said DeRosier told him he had a dream his grandmother died.

Testimony in his trial revealed he spoke openly to friends of his illogical hatred for his grandparents and especially his hatred of Ted Bieganek. One friend said DeRosier wanted his grandfather dead and that DeRosier said he wanted to be the man of the house. He took the friend through the house on one occasion. He told her the house would be his when his grandparents died.

A friend of Angie Bieganek testified DeRosier was told to bring the key for the house back on Christmas Eve and he was informed he could no longer do his laundry at his grandmother's house.

DeRosier grew up in a culture of alcohol. His parents owned a bar on one of the lakes in the area. His uncle owned a bar in a small community near Brainerd. The family's reputation was defined by the drinking and fighting that occurred in and around the bars and between factions. Visitors to the bar tell stories of the fights that would erupt with the DeRosiers bringing it on.

Alcohol was a part of his parent's life. His academic and social behaviors, his explosive anger, his school failure, his illogical thinking, and most critical, the inability to determine the consequences of his fixation on killing his grandmother to pay off his truck all fit the profile of prenatal exposure to alcohol.

On a late Sunday evening, less than a year later, police were called to an upstairs apartment above a bar in downtown Brainerd, Minnesota. Most of the action in this strip of night lights centered around patrons of the several bars that catered to the college students and crowds of locals on Friday and Saturday nights. Tourists had long since withdrawn from the lakes and were back in their city haunts. This Sunday night was an exception. This was not the common bar fight call. A fifteen year old teenager lay dead on the floor of the cheap upper floor apartment, shot in the chest, abdomen and upper arm.

I remember the moment I heard about the shooting. I was helping a neighbor pour his concrete driveway when a friend stopped by telling the news of the shooting. It seemed to be an open and shut case. A teenager went to an apartment to retrieve a stolen game. An argument ensued and the gun was pulled. When I heard the name of the shooter, I was not surprised.

He was a troubled kid. He had a history of behavioral problems.

His mother abandoned him, leaving him in the care of a violent father. Brain damage was evident in his low academic abilities and his anti-social, threatening, and violent behaviors He lived with his dad in a run down rental house in south east Brainerd, a house that was later condemned and torn down. A pit bull was his companion at home because his dad was not around very much.

Eventually he was enrolled in an intensive services program for EBD students. There, he challenged authority with physical threats until he left school and enrolled in Brainerd. He carried on his troubled life on the streets of Brainerd.

He had been one of my students. When he was at our school, there was a genuine fear he was a danger to teachers. He was one of the several students I had worked with over my career who I thought would either be dead or would kill someone by the age of twenty-one.

To look at him, you would not think he was a violent person. He was a good-looking young student, quiet and calm when he was doing what he wanted or could do, but would erupt with a deep violent quick threatening temper when a teacher would require him to do something he could not or did not want to do. His method of coping with his low academic levels was to erupt into threatened violence. He embodied the profile FASD and that of a school shooter, eventually lived up to that profile, only his shooting did not occur at a school.

Seventeen days later, the Brainerd Police Department was called to the same neon lit strip of bars, this time to investigate the disappearance of a 21 year old woman, last seen leaving the bar with a man well known to the officers. Erica Dahlquist quickly became a well-known name statewide, as the small mid-Minnesota city was galvanized into action searching for the missing woman. Soon the reality hit home and the searchers started looking for a body rather than trying to find Erica alive. Ponds were drained, searches parties looked along roads and wherever a body could possibly be hidden.

As time passed, the prime suspect, Billy Myears, confessed to the murder and was arrested. He was released when the evidence did not support his confession. The search for Erica stalled.

Finally, after seventeen long fruitless months and the announcement of a $50,000 reward from the Spotlight on Crime program with the Minnesota Department of Public Safety, the Crow Wing County Sheriff's department got a search warrant to search the wooded property of Myears' grandparents. During the search, a cadaver dog broke loose, and while searching for the dog, the dog handler found a shallow grave. Erica Dahlquist had been found. A day later, an arrest warrant was issued for Myears, who had skipped town with a carnival.

A nationwide search began for the 25 year old Myears. America's Most Wanted TV program profiled Myears. Ten minutes after the episode aired, a viewer in Michigan called the program and said she had recognized a tattoo on Myears when she saw him operating a Ferris wheel at a traveling carnival. This led to his capture. He pled guilty to second-degree murder and received a 250-month sentence.

Myears grew up on his grandfather's farm with his mother and siblings. His grandfather was well liked by neighbors, but according to sources, Myears' mother was considered "squirrelly" and exhibited alcoholic behaviors. She would leave the family for months at time, drinking and doing drugs, and then come home and dry out.

The slight farm boy had a troubled history in school as well as with the local authorities. He did not complete the seventh grade before he was placed in a highly restrictive behavioral management program. He was teased because he was in special classes. Other kids were mean to him because he had to wear dirty old clothes, presumably because his family was poor. He rarely saw his biological father. He had a litany of academic and social behavioral problems and dropped out of school after ninth grade. Adults who worked with him reported his ability to normally interact with others was minimal at best.

Myears had a criminal history. He had been charged with several misdemeanors, including trespassing, theft, disorderly conduct, and a fifth degree assault in which he was found guilty of threatening his sister and her boyfriend by showing them a clip to a handgun and threatening to use the gun on them. He was arrested for terroristic threats, but the charge was reduced to fifth degree assault and he was sentenced to 90 days in jail. Then October 30th came and Billy Myears moved from petty crimes to murder. Once again, this community was stunned by the actions of a man who fit the profile of prenatal exposure to alcohol.

The eighteen-month carnage was not done. On May 29, 2003, Cass County deputies raced to Pillager, a little community west of Brainerd, after receiving a murder report. The scene was bloody. Two bodies, a male and a female, lay in their own blood on the dirty floor of a shabby mobile home. The man had a gunshot wound to the head. The woman had been beaten to death. Outside, another man lay dead from a gunshot wound. Blood, large amounts of blood, was found in numerous areas throughout the death scene. All three deaths were ruled homicide.

Over two weeks later, Las Vegas Metropolitan Police Department detectives arrived at a seedy Las Vegas hotel to talk Benjamin Kennedy out of the room where he had barricaded himself. Kennedy had fled Minnesota after being charged with the three Pillager murders. Detectives had tracked him down to the squalid hotel. Throughout the day, negotiations continued, but failed, and finally the SWAT officers forced entry by kicking in the door and breaking the motel room's windows. Officers found him dead at the scene from a self-inflicted knife wound to the heart.

Benjamin Kennedy was born in Korea and was an adopted child. He grew up in Brainerd and attended the Brainerd schools. According to the *Brainerd Dispatch*, teachers in the Brainerd School District remembered him having difficulty in school. He was referred to and attended the alternative school because he was not doing well in high school. Kennedy dropped out as a senior.

Kennedy had ten years of history with the Cass and Crow Wing county court systems, having been charged with theft, driving under the influence, forging checks, carrying a gun without a permit, and disorderly conduct. He served a 15 month sentence for stealing two guns from a pawnshop. In August of that same year, DNA evidence linked Kennedy to the triple homicide.

While we will never know the irrational motive for the three slayings in Pillager, several factors in Benjamin Kennedy's life provide clues that point to the brain damage from prenatal exposure to alcohol. His social and academic behaviors as a student and behaviors as an adult fit the profile of prenatal exposure to alcohol. He was adopted, another factor that places him at a very high probability of prenatal exposure to alcohol. He had a disrupted school experience, had problems with drugs and alcohol, and was in trouble with the law, all factors that increase the probability of prenatal exposure to alcohol. When asked, his adopted father stated his son was most likely FAS.

In doing the research for this chapter, one aspect of the reporting became abundantly clear. The news reporting on Ben Kennedy, of Korean birth, included much more detail on his troubled life, including details of his educational struggles. When he committed the murders, he was an adult. DeRosier and Myears were treated with kid gloves compared to Kennedy. The fourth shooter is Native American, but was a juvenile when the event occurred, so I am giving the news reporting a break with him. Kennedy's father was right when he complained to me about the disparity in reporting and how his son was the target of racism in the Brainerd community.

The actions of the murderers during this dark period in the history of the Brainerd area are linked due to prenatal exposure to alcohol. Each of the men who committed the murders fits the profile of prenatal exposure to alcohol. Each exhibit behaviors of brain damage that contributed to their deviant, violent, illogical, abnormal thought processes, culminating in the death of seven innocent victims.

You say this isn't happening in your town? This is happening in your town and in every community, town, and city in this country. Our society is being strained by the aberrant, unreasonable, brutal thinking of a growing number of prenatally exposed boys and men. When accounts of violence appear in your local newspaper, ask those in authority this question: Was the accused exposed to alcohol before birth? If the answer is "We don't know," insist they find out.

CHAPTER Six

He Could Have Been a School Shooter

A s this book began to take shape, I had the opportunity to hear this story. I asked this mother to tell you her story, which is so familiar to me, as I have seen this type of behavior and the stressors in families due to FASD. This is a true story, and stories such as this are happening behind the scenes in your town. The names in this story have been changed to provide anonymity for the family.

A Mother's Story

I remember frantically calling my husband Joe to come home from work right away. Our thirteen-year-old son Michael was having one of his many episodes, but this time it was different. He had threatened to kill our family pet and me, and, at that moment, I believe he meant every word of it. Before I picked up Michael at school that day, I was concerned because he was angry all the time, wouldn't talk to us, and when not at school, he sat in his room in the dark. Earlier that day, I had decided it was time to look through his things to see if there were any clues to what was going on with him. Worried that drugs might be the culprit, instead I found a hunting knife and various switchblades hidden under clothing in his dresser. Additionally I found cigarette lighters and burned bits of paper and toothpicks hidden away in his room. I don't know where he got them, as they didn't belong to us, and we didn't give him money to buy such things. The combination of his depressed and angry state along with finding the weapons scared me out of my wits.

For months we had been attending family counseling to try to help him, but he wouldn't participate. He would just sit there and angrily glare at us throughout the sessions. My husband questioned why we were even going, asking how this was going to help if he's not wanting the help. Our son hated us, hated school, hated the kids at school, his teachers and administrators. He had many acquaintances at school, but no real friends because of his emotional and behavioral immaturity. Most other kids found him annoying at the very least. He was basically an outcast, shunned and teased by the very kids he strived to be with. He had nothing to lose, and had let anger and rage take over him. Michael was at the lowest point in his short life, and because of all of this, I feared he had the potential to become the next school shooter.

After finding the lighters and knives, I called his counselor, Kate, to see if we could get an emergency session. She was able to fit us in at 3:00 pm, which would mean pulling our son out of school a bit early. Kate told me not to tell him what I had found until we were in session because she needed to see his demeanor when answering as to why he had these things hidden in his room. I picked my son up and brought him home. He was pacing back and forth, angry, demanding I tell him what was going on. So I let him know that we had a counseling appointment but did not give him the details. "I don't want to go, you should have left me at school. I could KILL you!!!" Then he realized I had taken our pet chinchilla out of his room. She had lived in his room for years, but with his state of mind and upon finding the lighters and knives, I moved her into our bedroom and locked the door to keep her safe. He asked where she was and when I told him I moved her, he was screaming, throwing things, and trying to kick down our bedroom door, all the while threatening to kill her.

Years earlier, at age 7, Michael was under the care of a Pediatric Neurologist because of his behavior problems. He was diagnosed with ADD and prescribed Ritalin. When other more serious behaviors evolved, he was then diagnosed with Oppositional Defiant Disorder (ODD). Gradually, he was showing signs of depression and at the age of nine, he was prescribed Paxil to help with his depression. It wasn't long after starting his medication regiment when he described nightmares he was having about purposely setting our house on fire while we slept, then sneaking out of the house and leaving us all to burn to death. We took him off the Paxil and the nightmares went away. Finding the lighters, burned paper and toothpicks was even more frightening than finding the knives. At that point, he wasn't on any medication and hadn't been for some time.

When we arrived at Kate's office, Michael waited in the waiting room with Joe and our daughter while I spoke with her first. I had a brown paper bag filled with the knives, lighter, and burned items I had found. I told her about the threats our son had made and how terrified I was. She warned me there were a few choices as to what we were going to do about this and the choice would depend on his reaction and explanation about why the knives were in his room. The choice we were hoping for would have been for him to admit he needed help and participate in counseling. The other choices were to take him to a psychiatric hospital or call the police and have him arrested.

After hearing what I had to say, Kate called Michael and Joe to come in. She took the bag and dumped the items out on the table in front of Michael and asked him to tell her why he had these things. Michael sat silent; his eyes were full of rage. Next, she asked him if he had threatened to kill me. Michael tried to make light of the situation by suggesting I was crazy and that he didn't recall making a threat, but Kate pressed him further. She tried to make him understand if we didn't have an explanation for these things we found in his room, we would have to call the police because of the threat he made on my life. He just sat there and stared at all of us. Kate sent Michael back into the waiting room so she could talk with us. She said he was obviously depressed, and we should consider him dangerous to himself and to us. Her suggestion was to commit him to a psychiatric hospital.

There was no other choice, so we brought him to the emergency room, and waited for hours before anyone came in to see him. By the time the attending psychiatrist/physician came in to examine Michael, he was sleeping soundly on the exam table. Refusing to understand what we were dealing with, the doctor suggested since he was no longer angry or in a rage at that point, we should just take him home. I couldn't believe what I was hearing. We actually had to argue with the doctor, insisting we were not safe in bringing him home at that point and that he may be a danger to himself as well. The doctor finally relented and signed the authorization papers to have our son admitted to a psychiatric hospital.

Michael spent over two weeks there. He was diagnosed with Major Depression and put on Lexapro for depression and Strattera for his ADD. While he was in their care, our family had a much-needed break, as dealing with Michael's problems on a daily basis had taken quite a toll on all of us. Mostly, I used the time to catch up on some much needed sleep since up till that time I was barely sleeping at all so that I could stay up and make sure Michael wasn't doing something he shouldn't. I had to wait until he was asleep before I could sleep. Michael had insomnia and I got even less sleep than he did. I also took time to clean his room and make sure there were no weapons or unsafe items left in there. I also had Joe gather up all of his hunting rifles, shotguns and ammunition and get them out of the house, which he did. Until then, the guns were locked up, but that didn't seem like enough. If he really wanted something, Michael would find a way to get at it. Even if it meant waiting until we were asleep to get something he wanted, he could be quite devious. So the guns were taken to my in-laws' house about fifty miles away and were locked up there. I was still shaken up from having Michael threaten my life, so I also locked up the kitchen knives, scissors, anything sharp before he came home.

We started family counseling with Kate some months before when we realized Michael's behaviors and academic performance were quickly going downhill and he had run away from home one afternoon. We called all his friends, but no one knew where he was. Then we called the police when it got dark out and he still wasn't home. Some hours later, the police found him trying to enter his school for an activity night dance. Michael had been grounded for not doing homework and various other behaviors we were trying to stop. Whenever we gave him consequences, he became angry and rebellious to the point where he refused to be reprimanded and accept his consequences. He really wanted to go to the activity at school and nothing was going to stop him, not even the fact he was grounded already for other offenses, so he ran away.

Michael was also becoming very manipulative. He would always see himself as the victim even though clearly that was not the case. If his actions caused him to be grounded or lose privileges, he would blame us for his misfortune, rather than learning from his consequences and changing his behavior. He would tell lie after lie, even when there was no reason to lie. Lying became second nature for him, and he was very convincing about it.

Before we met with Kate the first time, I detailed in a letter all Michael's behavior problems, including the notes that came home, starting as early as kindergarten, telling of incidents where he couldn't sit still and pay attention and would excuse himself to go to the restroom. The teacher would inevitably notice he was missing for quite awhile, so she had to send someone in there after him. Michael was usually found climbing or running around the toilets, sinks and whatever else he could find to amuse himself. The notes also told of times when other students would report Michael because he was touching them and they did not want to be touched. This was usually poking people with his finger or tugging on their clothes. He would also talk incessantly, oblivious to the fact he was interrupting conversations or school lessons. The teacher would tell him to stop but he did not.

It was also around this time we found we had to "frisk" him whenever we were leaving someone's house, as he would "steal" various small objects (toys, keys, whatever) and stuff them in his pockets or break them and hide them somewhere. It didn't matter whose house, as Michael was not discriminatory, whether it be friends or family. When we would ask him why he did that, Michael would always reply, "I don't know." I was so frustrated with his conduct I found myself screaming at him, "If you don't know why you're going to do something, don't do it!" Screaming advice at him was a useless strategy as far as Michael was concerned.

As he grew older, his behavior became more serious. When

Michael was in second grade, his school principal called me on the phone, angrily conveying to me that my son had been throwing rocks on the playground during recess after being warned by a teacher. As soon as the teacher turned her back, Michael threw another rock and damaged a teacher's car. He was also refusing to do homework, and would instead tell me he had finished it in school. It got so bad his teacher had to call me every day to let me know what his homework assignments were, and I would do my best to get him to do them. Trying to teach him right from wrong proved impossible because he didn't seem to even care if there were consequences to his actions. Michael was basically grounded all the time, and those consequences never seemed to change his behavior.

By the time he reached third grade, we came to realize Michael was completely out of control. We had to leave him in the care of my parents because we were going to China to adopt our daughter and could not take him with. This was in the summer between grades, so Michael stayed at their house. My parents lived two blocks from my brother who has a son and a daughter near Michael's age. About a month after we returned, my sister-in-law informed me Michael had sexually molested her daughter while in my parent's care. We were in shock and could not figure out how he came to have such advanced sexual knowledge. My sister-in-law also called the police and Family Services in order to prosecute Michael. When questioned, Michael told police my niece initiated the sexual contact, but the police did not believe him since he was about a year older than my niece. Family Services got involved because they were concerned about the possibility of our son having been molested by an adult prior to this. Through investigation and required counseling, they found he had not been molested and labeled the case "unfounded."

Just prior to this event, my niece had been attending a home daycare run by an elderly couple. Later it was found the husband had been molesting the children in their care for years while the wife looked the other way and allowed it because they needed the income. This couple had gotten away with doing this for nine years before the molestations were brought to light and they were convicted. From reading books on this subject, I learned it is common for a child who has been molested to go on and molest other children. In that case, it appeared Michael was telling the truth, that our niece most likely initiated the contact from the experience she had in the daycare. We put Michael through some counseling as required by Family Services, and also explained he should not do this anymore because no one will let their kids play with him. Doing that with other kids was very bad, and if he did it again he might go to jail. We were trying to tell it to him in a way we hoped it would make an impression on him so he would not repeat what he had learned.

Unfortunately, nothing seemed to make an impression on Michael. Two years later, we discovered he had sexually molested a different female cousin, and this time it was definitely he who initiated it. Michael had no reservations about admitting what he did, and seemed confused as to why we were so upset about this. We brought Michael to my sister-in-law's house so we could all confront him about what he had done in the hopes it would be a wake up call for him when he realized the pain he had caused us all. My sister-in-law and I were crying. Michael sat there staring blankly. He showed absolutely no remorse. When asked why he would do such a thing after seeing all the pain we had gone through when this happened with our other niece, his reply was "I don't know."

Joe and I were terrified no matter how hard we tried to teach our son right from wrong, we may be raising a child molester or worse. There were times when I was driving somewhere with my son in the car, I actually considered driving off a bridge and killing us both. I didn't really want to die, but I didn't want to live through the torture of raising a man who lives to harm people. I reasoned if we could not help our son to change and live a positive life, then there was no point to him living either. I stopped short of carrying out such an act because I had a young daughter who needed me. Instead I desperately searched for help for our son until I found a therapist who specialized in Juvenile Sex Offender Therapy. I also told my doctor of what we were going through and the thoughts I was having. I was put on anti-depressants so I could handle the devastation that had become our lives.

Kate took some time to read the five-page letter outlining the horrors of our life with Michael. Afterwards, she asked "Michael was adopted, right?" and I said, "Yes", wondering if she was going to say his behaviors and emotional problems were due to something called

"Adopted Child Syndrome." I had heard of the term years ago, with claims adopted children with behavior problems or depression have these problems because they were separated from their birth family. Instead, Kate asked me if our son's birthmother drank alcohol while pregnant. I told her what I knew, that she wasn't an alcoholic, but a teenager who did drink alcohol a few times while pregnant and on at least two occasions she was drunk. Once was the night Michael was conceived, the other when his birthmother was in her 7th month of pregnancy. She was graduating high school and determined not to miss any parties. I asked her not to drink at the parties, but her response was she had earned it and she wasn't going to miss out. She also told me not to worry about the possibility of the baby being harmed because she didn't drink all the time so I had nothing to worry about. She also let me know in no uncertain terms, that just because she was carrying our future child did not give me the right to tell her what to do.

Kate then said our son most likely had Fetal Alcohol Effects (FAE), which was brain damage just the same as Fetal Alcohol Syndrome, but without the easy-to-diagnose facial features. Up till then, I had thought only alcoholic women put their babies at risk of FAS. Kate told us about new studies and information that were showing a few drinks at the wrong time during a pregnancy could cause brain damage and behavioral problems just like we were seeing in Michael. I asked her to tell us everything she knew about FAE. We wanted to know where to take him for a diagnosis. We needed to know what it meant for his future. We needed to know how to help him. Was there a cure? Unfortunately, she had nothing to offer, all she seemed to know was Michael's behavior patterns and learning problems were classic symptoms of FAE.

Finding there was a possible reason behind our son's behavior problems and he wasn't choosing to be this way was somewhat of a relief. It also helped to know we were not responsible for Michael's conduct. As his parents, we were under pressure from school officials to get his behavior under control. Much of our family did not understand our son's behaviors and accused us of not being vigilant in watching him or handing out punishment. Some members of my husband's family even left our kids out when inviting the rest of the entire family for gatherings such as weddings and anniversary parties, and friends stopped calling to get together. We had spent the first thirteen years of our son's life trying everything we could to change him, all to no avail. We tried grounding him and taking away privileges. When that didn't work we tried shaming him, lectures, and spanking him when the more humane types of punishment didn't work. Just as kids at school shunned our son, friends and family shunned us because of Michael's behavioral challenges.

Since Kate had no resources for us to learn about this disorder she called Fetal Alcohol Effects, I knew it was up to me to educate myself on the subject. I checked with our local library, but they had no current books on the subject. The Internet turned out to be my best source of information. I found books, support groups, medical facilities that did diagnostics and a plethora of information on the subject. First I learned FAE was no longer the term used to describe the disorder, instead the term "Fetal Alcohol Spectrum Disorders" was used to describe the varying levels of damage caused by prenatal exposure to alcohol, and there were different labels within that spectrum that defined the specific type of damage.

Another thing I learned was a high percentage of identified individuals with Fetal Alcohol Spectrum Disorders (FASD) are adopted. That fact was supported in evidence by the support group of parents raising adult children with FASD I had joined. In the more than 100 parents in our online group there are only a few who are biological parents, the rest are adoptive parents. People might think most of these children are Native American or from places like Russia where FASD runs rampant. However many of these young adults with FASD were born to birthparents who were non-Native American US citizens. It does stand to reason many babies who become available for adoption in the US are born to teenagers who are not ready to parent, such as in Michael's case. It is the worst possible time for young women to get pregnant since they are not only experimenting with sex, but usually with alcohol, so the fact many adopted children in the US have FASD is not really all that surprising.

The high incidence of FASD in adopted children and the similarity in behavioral problems, impulsivity and learning disabilities led me to believe the term "Adopted Child Syndrome" (ACS) was actually FASD all along. Back when the term ACS was first used, it was not known moderate or occasional binge drinking by a mother could cause brain damage and these types of symptoms. The assumption was made that being adopted had some lasting psychological effect, even though many of these children were adopted at birth and had no knowledge or memory of their birth family.

A few weeks shy of his seventeenth birthday, Michael was finally diagnosed with ARND (alcohol related neuro-developmental disorder), which is brain and neurological damage caused by prenatal exposure to alcohol. He was also diagnosed with Dysthymic Disorder, which is being in a chronic state of depression for more than 2 years. The doctors had many recommendations to help with his school IEP and transition into adulthood. By then he was refusing to take medication and he knew once he turned seventeen, we could not force him to take medication since he was considered an adult and had the right to make his own choices. For some time, he had been planning on leaving home when he turned seventeen because he also knew we could not have the police find him and bring him home. He refused to live by any rules we had and he refused to accept any consequences given to him because of his disobedience.

From the time we learned about FASD and came to understand its effect on Michael, we tried to alter our methods of parenting based on his lack of understanding consequences. We lowered our expectations of him and realized he was doing the best he could, even though to others it was hard to believe. We tried to focus on his good qualities, which at that point were very hard to see, as he had pretty much shut down emotionally, academically and otherwise. We praised him when we were able, but it was too late by then. After years of struggling and having everyone around him not understand his challenges and behavior problems, he had given up.

On his seventeenth birthday, Michael moved out of our home. He had made plans to move in with the Boyd family. The Boyds have four sons who were frequently in trouble with the law and the family was in need of rent money. Their family was split up with two sons living with their mom, and two sons living with the dad in separate residences. Michael was a friend of all of their sons. There was little in the way of rules or structure in their homes, everyone pretty much did whatever they wanted there, and that appealed to Michael. They felt sorry for him because he had them believing we were extremely strict, and we were standing in the way of letting him make his own decisions. It's true we had to supervise him constantly, and had rules in place for him most of his friends did not have, mainly because of his poor judgment and lack of understanding right from wrong. He also had the Boyds believing we had kicked him out of our house on his seventeenth birthday so they couldn't say "No" to letting him move in. The mom, Patty, had Michael agree to go to work with her sons some weeknights after school and weekends so he could afford to pay rent. He also had to agree to stay in school.

For the first month or so he lived with Patty and the two boys who lived with her. It didn't take long for Michael to renege on his end of the deal. He would go to school for a few hours then cut out. He would also get into arguments with one of the sons. Patty told him he couldn't stay there any longer. The sons were living with the father felt sorry for him, so they talked the dad into letting Michael move in there, though he would have to work part time, pay rent, and go to school. Michael agreed, but instead he would stay up all night playing video games or going on the Internet, and of course, be too tired to go to school. He was not bathing regularly and did not wash his clothes. He brought friends in who sometimes stole things from the people he was living with. He would make excuses so he didn't have to go to work and subsequently didn't have the money to pay the rent he had promised. At the time, Michael had a girlfriend who suffered mental and emotional problems. They had a very volatile relationship. Instead of normal conversations, they would often get into arguments that turned into non-stop screaming, and the neighbors would call the police. Michael and his girlfriend would often cut school and go to the house when no one was home. He was also going out drinking all night and would get into knife fights.

While Michael lived with the Boyds, I would try to check on him to make sure he was all right. He resented my attempts to contact him if the family was around because he wanted them to believe we had kicked him out so he could continue living there. The first couple of times I went there, he flat out told me to leave. When I tried calling, he wouldn't answer, or he would hang up on me. Other times, he would call to taunt me and say things like "Hey mom, guess what – I'm DRUNK!!" At the time, Michael's school was still in contact with us because we were still legally responsible for his welfare and his IEP. The school was aware of Michael's current living arrangements, and they were concerned because of his frequent absences, his poor hygiene, and the fact they noticed he hadn't been eating properly and had lost weight. Michael was also either sleeping in class or refusing to participate. He would get into verbal confrontations with the teachers, then storm out of the classroom.

The school administration was sympathetic. They understood there wasn't much that we could do to change things, but they warned us they were required to report the situation to the Department of Children and Family (DCFS) services because if Michael's poor health, hygiene, and state of mind continued or worsened, they could be held responsible for neglecting to report it. In spite of the fact that they had to report it, it appeared the school administration did not want us to be in trouble, so they suggested if we gave Michael money for food/clothing, we would not be held responsible for Michael's current state. In theory, that might have sounded reasonable, except if we handed Michael money, he would not have used it for food or clothing or for doing his laundry. Instead, he would have used it to buy alcohol, cigarettes, and other things he shouldn't be buying. Handing him money would have made a bad situation even worse, and that was out of the question. We were also holding out hope that without monetary support from us to continue his insane lifestyle, Michael would give up and come home.

At that point, we were between a rock and a hard place. I decided to call one of his friends and plead with them to get Michael to talk to me. I told the friend because of what Michael was doing, we may be investigated by DCFS and it was not fair to do that to us as we were still raising his sister, and we feared they might take her away. Within a few hours Michael called me. We talked about the school's concerns and I told him he was welcome to come home for dinner every day if he wanted to since he only lived about a mile away. I also offered to buy him some clothing. He still didn't want to bother coming to our house to eat, so a few times a week, I would bring him leftovers so he had something to eat, since he wasn't always paying the rent like he had agreed, and the Boyds couldn't afford to feed him. Michael had been living with the Boyds a total of five months when he called me to ask if he could move back home. It was not because he came to his senses. The Boyds were fed up with police being called, Michael bringing strange people in their house, the drinking, the fights, and most importantly, no rent coming in; they were kicking him out.

I can't say we were overjoyed at the prospect of our son returning home. Living with him was difficult before he moved out, and he would no doubt be even more difficult to control after having all the freedom to do whatever he wanted for the months he was living with the Boyds. Before he returned, Joe and I made up a contract, carefully listing all the rules he had to agree to live by if he wanted to move back in. We told him if he did not follow the rules, he would have to leave. Michael resentfully signed the contract. For a while, Michael followed most of the rules. The few minor rules he broke were dealt with by consequences such as losing his TV privileges for a few days or something similar. We had also told Michael if he could not follow most of the rules and at least make an effort to show us some respect, then we would have to bring him to a homeless shelter. We just couldn't go on living like that anymore.

During this time, Michael stayed in school, however it was more of a place to go for social interaction rather than learning. In spite of his IEP, high school was torture for our son. His teachers and IEP manager did not understand his type of brain damage or how it affected his ability to learn. They also didn't understand his rebellious ways and frustration in the classroom. They wanted to focus on the fact he has ADD when that was the least of his problems. I went to every IEP meeting and tried to explain to them what I had learned about FASD and how it affected Michael. He could sometimes learn things, but with the brain damage he had, he would "forget" where he stored the information he had learned. He would complete some homework assignments and it would appear he had a fair understanding of the work he was doing; but if given a test on the same material sometime later, he would completely flunk the test. This was because he could not recall the information he had previously learned.

His IEP meetings were somewhat of a joke. Michael's IEP team which included teachers, a social worker, counselor, and principal, absolutely refused to take the time to learn about FASD which would have helped them learn how to teach my son, what to expect of him, what not to expect, and it would have shown them Michael was not in control of his behavior, so to punish him for it as they would a "normal" student was futile and further degrading. Out of desperation I purchased a bunch of copies of the book "Damaged Angels" which was written by Bonnie Buxton, a woman whose adopted daughter had the same diagnosis of "ARND" as our son Michael. Her daughter's struggles, challenges, and behaviors were very similar to our sons. I took the books to an IEP meeting and explained this would help them not only learn about my son and how to teach him, but would help them understand his behaviors. I also told them he is not likely the first kid with FASD to enter their school system, and by statistics, he will not be the last, so they wouldn't only be helping my son, but others by learning about FASD. I handed one book to my son's IEP manager and another to his social worker. His IEP manager rolled her eyes and made excuses as to why she didn't have the time to read it but took the book anyway. The social worker was a bit more gracious, as he thanked me and said it looked "interesting" though I have no idea if he actually read it.

Since his freshman year, they all decided Michael was "smart enough" to take pre-algebra. At first, Michael tried to keep up, but was only able to manage for about two weeks. This was because the first two weeks were spent reviewing what he had managed to learn back in grade school. After that, the abstract concepts of Algebra were lost on Michael, he tried a little longer but eventually he gave up and failed. Once again, in his second year of high school they insisted on putting him back in pre-algebra. I argued the point with his IEP manager and literally begged them to put him in the simplest math class they could. His IEP manager argued back that he was "smart enough", and I was underestimating his abilities, and there was no reason he couldn't do this if he really wanted to. In her opinion he was failing because he was lazy and didn't do most of the homework. She also insisted if he were given basic math, he would get bored, and Basic Math wouldn't prep him for college. COLLEGE?!!! This kid couldn't even pass high school classes, and they were insisting he had to prep for college. This time they were putting him in a class with a different teacher, who had an assistant teacher there to help learning disabled students. The results were the same, and Michael once again failed. In his third year, again they put him in Pre-Algebra. This time he didn't even try because he knew what the outcome was going to be, so why bother?

Algebra was Michael's worst subject in high school, but that is not to say he didn't have difficulty in other subjects. He had a hard time retaining things he had read, so any class that required reading something and remembering what he read was difficult for him. He had teachers call him "Stupid." Other times he would ask the same question more than once because he didn't understand something about material they were covering, and if he asked the same question more than once, he was accused of being high. He was not "high", he really needed to ask the questions.

Because of his ARND, which also causes social immaturity, Michael had a difficult time relating to other students in school. The only social circles he seemed welcome in were groups of other troubled teens. Occasionally he would become friends with a non-troubled teen, but those relationships usually didn't last very long, as it wouldn't take long for those kids to tire of Michael's immaturity and manipulating ways. What made it worse was being labeled as "learning disabled." He felt the "normal" kids all thought he was retarded.

Michael would often play the part of a "Class Clown" or "Class Bad Ass" in order to gain acceptance. In classes where he was required to do a speech, he would get stressed out and cut school or become physically ill because he did not want to get up in front of everyone and have his intelligence, or lack thereof, judged by his peers. When one such speech was coming up, I could see Michael becoming more and more agitated as the deadline grew near, I asked the teacher if he could possibly work on a different project on the same subject that wouldn't require him to get up in front of the class, but she refused. In the end, Michael just refused to do it and accepted a failing grade instead.

When I finally had our son's ARND diagnosis on paper, I went in to Michael's IEP meeting and showed them the recommendations that were made to help my son learn. For the past couple of years, Michael would purposely get into trouble in order to be put into something the school calls "Isolation"(ISO). This was a form of in-school suspension where the few kids who had ISO were put in individual cubicles set up near the principal's office to do their schoolwork. There was always at least one teacher there to supervise and help out with any questions they may have had. Michael did very well under those circumstances, as he had the peace and quiet he needed to get work done and he was able to focus and concentrate. There the lights weren't as bright as in the classroom and people weren't moving around and talking all the time. During a prior meeting, Michael asked if he could be in "Isolation" every day, as he knew he functioned better under those conditions. He was told he could not, as their reasoning was they didn't have the resources to provide that kind of environment for him on an everyday basis and they had to reserve space in ISO for kids who were given ISO as consequences.

It so happened when his diagnosis for ARND was done, the assessment found Michael also had sensory processing difficulties, meaning he gets over stimulated and agitated when certain things like background noise, bright lights and such overload his senses. Sensory processing difficulties are common in people who have ARND and other Fetal Alcohol Spectrum Disorders. The report suggested Michael learn in a quiet area with less traffic and light. I mentioned that in the IEP meeting, to inform them why "Isolation" worked so much better for Michael, and I asked them to reconsider the possibility of letting him utilize "Isolation" for most of his classes. They refused and told me doing so would be counter productive because he needed to learn to socialize properly and to not be a loner.

The IEP team refused to understand they were never going to get him to learn effectively under the current circumstances. They were blind to what his true challenges were. The IEP team members were so insistent on doing things their way and shutting me out that they whipped out a contract for me to sign, stating I understood I would no longer be notified of Michael's upcoming IEP meetings when he turned eighteen. He had just turned seventeen, and they were asking me to sign this a full year before he turned eighteen! I never yelled or threatened in an IEP meeting, I was just there to make suggestions to help them find a way to successfully teach my son. Looking back, I realize they allowed me to be there because they had to; however, they really did not want to hear what I had to say and had no intention of following any advice.

In the fall of 2006, a young man named Eric Hainstock shot and killed the principal of his high school in Cazenovia, Wisconsin. Eric was known as a troubled student with learning disabilities, much like my son. We live in northern Illinois, near the Wisconsin border, so this one was very close to home. The day after this happened, my son's IEP team had a meeting, which they did not invite me to. I believe they did not label it an "IEP" meeting because they would have been required to notify me of the meeting in advance so I could be there. When finished with their meeting, they called me on the phone and asked me to persuade my son drop out of school immediately, as they had decided he "did not want to be there." This was during the time when my son was living with the Boyd family. The school knew my son was living completely unsupervised, and no one really knew if he had access to any weapons. He would look for any reason to get into a confrontation with certain teachers so he could mouth off at them and then storm out of the room, only to spend the day in the principal's office. To my understanding, some of his teachers feared him, and I had heard some requested Michael be transferred to someone else's class.

Apparently they recognized the very real threat of my son's state of mind. I knew dropping out at that point was out of the question for Michael, as his agreement with the Boyds stipulated he could only live in their home if he was going to school full time because they did not want him hanging around their house all day with his friends. Besides, as a mother, I was still holding out hope things would change and allow for my son to get the type of education he needed, but that was not to be.

By May of his junior year in high school, Michael had been back living in our home for five months after being kicked out of the Boyds house in December. Even though he stayed in school (per our rules) he was failing most of his classes. He had completely shut down in school and was accomplishing nothing apart from aggravating or scaring the school faculty. He was also refusing to see a doctor and start on medication again. Then one day he disappeared. I tried calling his friends and no one seemed to know where he was. After about two weeks, he finally called me and told me he had been living in another state with one of the Boyd boys. Michael also said he was going to come home to get his things and live somewhere in town with friends. He did pick up his things and was gone a few more days when he called and asked if he could move home again because he had nowhere to go. I again reminded him of the rules and that he had to agree to abide by them. He also announced he was done with trying to finish school. He was dropping out.

One of our house rules had been he had to stay in high school until he graduated. By this time, I realized Michael had nothing left in him to keep going in school. The lack of cooperation from his IEP team convinced me this was a losing battle, and I just couldn't force Michael to endure it anymore. He had decided to drop out of high school, and at this point, I agreed with him, insisting he would have to get his GED. Unfortunately, our laws state that someone cannot get their GED until their graduating class has graduated. This law was in place so they don't have kids dropping out of school left and right to "take the easy way out." Michael had been held back in 8th grade for an extra year because we decided he wasn't ready for high school. The kids he went all through school with just graduated this year, but since Michael was held back in 8th grade, his graduating class was changed to add another year.

In the years raising my son, I would sometimes depend on my mom for emotional support. My mother kept reminding me she put the "mother's curse" on me because my behavior was out of control when I was Michael's age. She said, "Someday you will have a child just like you", and I did just that. Although my son is adopted, he is very much like me. I had difficulties in school especially in algebra; I also have ADD, which was not diagnosed until I grew up. I used drugs, cut school, I couldn't handle money, I stole from my mother's purse, I had very poor judgment, was depressed and full of rage. I barely graduated from high school and made it through only because I was in a diversified program that sent me to beauty school for half the school day in my junior & senior years. Then, with only one hundred and two hours left to graduate beauty school, I dropped out. I was having sex by the age of 14, and by the age of 18, had become promiscuous.

I also made very poor choices, and at one point I was engaged to a man who was in prison for the murder for hire of his wife. I met him after his wife was dead, but before anyone knew he had been responsible for her death. I stayed in that long distance, futile relationship for two years because I had no self-esteem, and I had found the only person on earth who actually made me feel needed instead of worthless. I got into a lot of trouble with my parents because I didn't understand the value of having rules. Even though I was given consequences, I would make the same mistakes over and over. My rages and behavior angered my father so much that he used to beat me to try to get me under control, which did not work. Instead it made me angrier and I would fantasize about killing him in his sleep because no matter what I did, it was never right and never good enough and he let me know quite often.

When I brought my son in for diagnosis, it finally dawned on me to ask my mother if she drank alcohol while she was pregnant with me. "Not THAT much" she said, referring to the fact my son's teenaged birthmother binge drank to the point she was drunk sometimes while pregnant with him. My mother drank socially during monthly card games with her friends (two to three drinks), or at the occasional party while pregnant with me. Because of this, I believe I too have FASD, but not as severe as my son. I also believe it's possible my prenatal exposure rendered me infertile. I went through menopause at the age of 20. After many tests including exploratory laparoscopic surgery, and chromosome analysis, the doctors couldn't find the cause. They said, "This was a birth defect, you were born with many fewer eggs than you should have had. This was likely due to something your mother was exposed to while pregnant with you." Well, the only thing I know I was exposed to was alcohol and cigarettes in utero. I also know with prenatal exposure to alcohol, the alcohol will damage whatever is forming in the baby at the time the alcohol is drunk. Alcohol is known to damage the brain, but also internal organs and the formation of facial features and extremities, so why wouldn't it damage the reproductive system if that were forming while alcohol was being consumed? It makes perfect sense to me.

In addition to premature menopause, I have a variety of other disorders or deformities. I have flat feet and obstructive sleep apnea. When I was younger, I was bulimic for years. Currently I am overweight and cannot seem to get my eating habits under control. I have had varying degrees of depression, and have at times been suicidal. I have been on medication for depression much of my adult life, and the times I was not, I probably should have been. I don't know if all of these disorders are related to my mom having consumed alcohol while pregnant with me, but I think it's worth mentioning. More is being learned everyday about FASD and its effects, so I believe it's entirely possible they will find more even problems are linked to prenatal exposure to alcohol.

My mom had a group of friends who were all pregnant at one time or another in the late 50's and early 60's. They got together at card games at least once a month and drank alcohol, whether they were pregnant or not. At the time, they were led to believe a couple of drinks wouldn't hurt the baby. Some of their children also had major behavioral problems, learning difficulties, and in their teens, trouble with the law.

Among these six women, one woman has a son with bi-polar disorder and had severe behavioral problems when growing up; another of her sons also had behavioral problems and depression. One of mom's friends has a son who was diagnosed with schizophrenia as an adult. During his early teens through twenties, he had some frightening behaviors and spent time in a psychiatric hospital. She also had a second son with ADD, and her daughter battled depression for years and tried to commit suicide. When she was in eighth grade, she spent some time in a psychiatric hospital. Another one of my mom's friends has a son who is mentally disabled and aimlessly wanders around the country. His mother has to find him to get his disability money to him. Another of the mothers who consumed alcohol when pregnant has a daughter, who had comprehension difficulties in school, has a congenital hole in her heart, Shogren's disease, flat feet and infertility issues. Another friend had 4 children, most if not all, had varying degrees of learning and/or behavioral problems. Two of them had teen pregnancies. The sixth is my mother. She had me with my aforementioned problems and my brother who has learning disabilities, behavioral problems, drug addiction, money problems, and ADD. Our sister doesn't appear to have learning disabilities, but she has physical problems such as fibromyalgia, was anorexic when in high school, and she is very moody. This seems like an extraordinarily high ratio of children with challenges for six friends and mothers. The obvious undeniable common denominator is prenatal exposure to alcohol.

I grew out of the negative behaviors somewhere in my mid 20's. However, I still struggle with poor organization, ADD and depression. I have never been able to hold a full time job without excessive absences and have lost jobs because I wasn't "productive enough." Basically they were telling me I worked too slowly. I do need extra time to gather my thoughts and that hurts my job performance reviews. I am also fortunate my husband is able to support us, so my income is just to help out. If I had to support our family, I don't think I could handle that.

It's hard to imagine how Michael will fare, being a male in our society; he would be expected to support a family. So far, he has had five jobs, none of which lasted longer than two weeks. The main reason for losing his jobs is his immaturity, low productivity, and poor memory. When he lost those jobs, he became frustrated and blamed his bosses or co-workers. I fear if this pattern of job loss and frustration continues, he may lose what little control he has and some day "go postal." He is like an eight year old in the body of an eighteen year old. Michael has goals and dreams, but does not understand how to carry through on them. We try to guide him, but he says he has to learn his way and he becomes angry when we try to give him advice. Without any support he is very likely to end up as a FASD statistic – homeless, in prison, on drugs, or dead. Even with support he will have an extremely difficult life.

In a follow-up email conversation with this struggling mother, I was struck by the honesty she portrayed.

You are a brave woman! I am humbled and honored to have your powerful story in the book.

To which she replied:

I never thought of myself as brave. Some of the things I wrote in the chapter about my life when I was younger, I have never even told my husband about for fear of what he would think. I do feel it's important to be brutally honest about those things in the chapter because it shows a contrast between how FASD affects males and how it affects females. Males with FASD tend to be more aggressive and outwardly destructive (FASD + testosterone = violence), while females with FASD are more emotionally vulnerable and tend to self-destruct. That's why I thought it was important to add a description of my behaviors, so people who read the book wouldn't be wondering why, if FASD was the reason for many of the shootings, why girls weren't shooting up the schools as well.

Coincidentally, the man I was engaged to who was in prison for the murder-for-hire of his wife, I believe he and his sister likely have FASD. Their father was an alcoholic, and their mother, though maybe not alcoholic, did like to drink. His motive for having his wife killed was money, mainly because their home had flooded and there was so much damage it was uninhabitable and it had not been insured, on top of that, he had trouble managing money, was addicted to drugs and he was physically abusive to his wife and didn't want to pay child support (which I found out later). His sister was also a drug addict, who around the time of her brother's wife's murder, committed insurance fraud on her house which also was nearby in the flood area. She got her ex-husband to agree to torch the house for a cut in the insurance money. He made a mistake and caused a gas explosion, got burned, and subsequently arrested. The sister died of a drug overdose about 15 years ago.

She is living the life where the abnormal has been her normalcy, where every waking moment of the day is impacted by prenatal exposure to alcohol, a life that could have been so different if the birth mother had not drank during the pregnancy.

This mother asked if I could examine a picture of her son to see if I could recognize any physical features of FAS. After looking at his picture, I could not. He is a fine looking young man. He is one of the 70% or more of brain damaged children whose face hides the damage. Anyone who does not have any knowledge of this young man's brain damage or understanding of brain damage behaviors from prenatal exposure to alcohol would look at him and think he thinks like any other person his age and should act as such.

Unfortunately, he can't. His is the face of the hidden epidemic.

His emotional age is much less than his actual age. His thinking will continue to confound those around him, eventually landing him in serious trouble. He will need someone to be his financial brain, his behavioral brain, and his emotional brain, but he will only find that support from his mother and only if he accepts that support. Others think he looks normal and that his actions are willful.

He will not be emancipated from adult care for many years, if ever. When he was young, his parents provided structure in his life. When he was in school, the school officials and teachers gave him some structure. Now, that is gone. If he does not have his mother or another adult acting as his "seeing eye brain," or "external brain", there is a good chance he will break the law and the judicial system will become his adult caregiver. Our jails are filled with men with similar brain damage.

Few young men with his level of brain damage successfully find a long-lasting mate. His illogical, immature, and potentially violent behaviors will eventually drive prospective mates away. Keeping a job will be difficult. Managing money will be a lifetime struggle. Testosterone raging through a young man's body is hard to control with a healthy brain. With his brain damage, he will have significant trouble managing his sexual life. His mother has already witnessed his screaming relationship with his girlfriend. His future relationships have the potential of physical abuse and worse.

She loves her son, but she knows the future. Hers is the plight of many adoptive and biological mothers of prenatally exposed boys, even if the mothers are in denial. Her life is consumed with the worry of who will be his adult caregiver. I know who will.

Taxpayers.

CHAPTER Seven
The Perfect Storm

"He's got a gun!" she quietly spoke in the phone. I took the phone call from a teacher who had just stepped off a bus full of students. "He got on the bus without me noticing, and I heard a gun. I heard something that sounded like a gun." The teacher kept her wits about her this crisp fall day in 1993, and when the bus stopped at its destination, she calmly guided the students into the building without raising any alarm.

The seventh grade student she identified could change the environment of the school through violent actions. He had been suspended from school and was not to be at any school function. Since our school was in the middle of the community, he had snuck into the line of students entering the bus without being noticed by the staff. He had a history of deviant behaviors, including coming to the school so drunk he could hardly walk, ending up on the staff bathroom floor. There were times he was fun to be with and seemed to want to do the best he could. We did not know which personality he would present at any given time or any given day. We were always on watch when he was in the school.

On a previous occasion, I had to take him home after he had been suspended for one of his many transgressions. The common knowledge in the community led me to believe I would not find his unemployed parents at home. I drove up to the dilapidated windblown house and had to kick the beer cans away from the door in order to get near enough to knock. He moved past me into the sparsely furnished house. I could see this was not where he would want to be. School was where he could be in warm place and have good meals. No wonder he wanted to be with the students when he was suspended, rather than be relegated to staying home.

His reputation gave me alarm as I rushed to the scene with urgency never before felt. By the time I slid to a stop in front of the building, all the students had filed into the large assembly room without knowing we knew he had a gun. He was quietly moved to a separate hallway to wait for me. The adults were safely out of the line of fire around a corner as I entered the building. He stood slouched against the wall, hood up and hands in his sweatshirt pockets. For the first time in my career, I felt the tightening of fear in my belly. My history with him gave me pause as to how to handle this situation. We had called the police, but our experience with the tribal police gave me cause to take care of this possible weapon as soon as possible.

He averted his eyes as I moved close to him. "What do you have?" I asked. His hand dipped into his zippered hooded sweatshirt. The tension was palpable, but I was not going to show any fear. His hand slowly drew a heavy, silver, automatic pistol, and he raised his eyes to mine. I did not move, waiting for his move. He slowly handed the weapon to me, and it was not until I had the pistol in my hands that I realized it was a replica of an automatic large caliber pistol with a functioning trigger and hammer. Within minutes, the tribal police chief arrived at the scene, took the juvenile into custody, and then promptly released him without any charges.

Within months, I experienced the second look-alike weapon. Our new school had only been open less than a year and already we had two weapons incidents and no weapons policy. A female student, angry with her teacher, knocked on her classroom door before the school day started. When the newly licensed female teacher opened the door, she was staring down the muzzle of a pistol, held by an arrogant, insolent juvenile girl. The student laughed it off and ridiculed the teacher for showing fear. The teacher had nightmares from this incident and soon left our school for a safer environment. The student was charged with the incident and left our school.

Our most frightening weapons incident was caught on camera. We had established a highly restrictive behavioral program within our main building. We needed to provide a safe environment for our students who needed a highly structured setting. Every corner of the room was covered with our surveillance cameras. Students were very aware of this fact. Video clips were used as deterrents, in meetings with parents, and in court when needed. Every physical interaction with students was sent to me for review as a way of monitoring staff and student actions.

A shocked and angry staff person called me to the program classroom. The tone and tenor of his voice immediately raised an alarm in my mind. I raced to the room, where he was sitting as if he had been knocked in the head. He directed me to the video where I watched in horror as one of his students walked up to him from behind, placed a derringer to his head, and pulled the trigger. You could see the teacher's body jump with fear as he realized what had happened. Staff rushed to disarm and subdue the student. The tribal police were immediately called. A look-alike derringer, indistinguishable from a real gun on the video, was the weapon of choice for this student. Once again, we had dodged the real thing. The question remained, when would we have a real shooter?

The potential shooter detailed first in this chapter continued his criminal career, going on a crime spree with an adult from a near-by city, doing a home invasion, kidnapping and sexually assaulting a young female victim, and ending up in a juvenile placement for sexual predators. His younger brother, while a fourth grade student, lit a female teacher's hair on fire. His younger sister was so impacted by prenatal exposure to alcohol she will never live independently.

Our second and third potential school shooters had academic and behavioral characteristics of FASD. The grandmother of the third potential shooter confirmed he was a victim of his mother's drinking. He was adjudicated to juvenile detention and later continued his life of crime until he was incarcerated as an adult.

The Storm of Factors

I believe the weapon events at this school were each committed for different reasons, known only to the perpetrators, but originated from a whirlwind of factors in each child's life. Each of these potential shooters lived in a chaotic home with little or no parental guidance. Each had identified disabilities that heavily impacted their everyday academic life. Each had a history of alcohol abuse, and all were children of alcoholic mothers. Each would be described as a troubled child. All exhibited behavioral characteristics of FASD.

The FASD brain can't realistically and logically deal with the realities of adolescence. Adolescent kids are socially brutal to each other at times, especially when adults are not around. Any physical difference can lead to unbearable teasing or bullying. Adults, both at home and at school, who should be the protectors of students, use shaming and blaming language that can further scar the FASD brain and thrust the child into depression. Academic failure further isolates the brain-damaged child, a child who already has difficulty interacting with peers.

Individuals with brain damage have little or no resiliency, the ability to handle stressful situations and respond more positively to difficult events. When mitigating factors in their lives trigger an emotional response, an FASD brain does not react the way we expect a brain should react.

To help people understand the concept of specific brain damage, I use a "blind spots" analogy to illustrate the specific parts of the brain that are damaged, leaving the thinking process flawed. Depending on the level of damage, any number of blind spots will be evident through some type of behavior. An academic behavior exhibited by the inability to remember multiplication facts, for instance, reveals a blind spot in the hypocampus. The inability to understand personal cues, the normal non-verbal language of human beings, reveals a blind spot in the frontal lobes. Combinations of blind spots are revealed through behaviors.

The potential shooters I personally dealt with had blind spots, that rigid, unresilient thought process, an obvious lack of judgment, the inability to understand the consequences of their actions, the frustrating, maddening, frightening incapability of logically organizing and self-monitoring their thoughts to stop the journey down the path to violence.

I call this whirlwind of factors the "Perfect Storm." Not all factors are easily preventable and most occur without adults knowing, understanding, or caring about the situations that bring on the factors in the Perfect Storm. I believe the first, and for the most part unknown and most significant factor, is an FASD brain with a lethal combination of "blind spots" in the brain.

An FASD brain under stress will display behaviors unlike a normal brain, for example, a violent illogical outburst followed by a remorseful apology and a promise it won't happen again, only to have the same outburst happen again, without regard to consequence, even when punitive action had been served. Blind spots in judgment, in understanding personal cues, in understanding consequences, in moral judgment, in emotional control, in impulse control are all evidence of brain damage. And these blind spots do not act in isolation. The combination of brain damage prohibiting the potential shooter's brain resiliency is the lethal factor most overlooked in the research of school shooters and criminals throughout our society.

The second most powerful factor is a school experience that traumatizes the FASD brain. The FASD "Perfect Storm" brain does not have the resiliency to ignore bullying and teasing by peers. **School teachers and administrators who use a punitive discipline policy system with shaming and blaming language or who refuse to understand the behaviors are a result of brain damage drive the FASD brain toward depression, anger, rebellion, and ultimately, a disrupted school experience and trouble with the law.**

Don't Be Fooled

Some school shooters across the nation were classified as "honor students" or good students. I have been an educator long enough to know these terms can be deceptive. Students with a Special Education Individual Education Plan could have all A's and be on the Honor Roll and be rightly considered an Honor Student. The same student may not be able to read anywhere near their chronological age level or may possess other characteristics of brain damage that is displayed in social behaviors more than academic behaviors.

I have also worked with enough prenatally exposed children to know some have exceptional intelligence along with lack of judgment, lack of impulse control, and/or other behaviors of brain damage. Many times, some of the brain damage behaviors are masked by medication. As stated before, FASD victims have scored 140 on IQ tests. They also have scored outside the norm on behavioral scales. The ethanol in the alcohol does not choose what damage to do, the amount and timing of exposure creates the opportunity for the ethanol to do its damage. A child exposed one time with one binge, at a certain time during the pregnancy, may only suffer brain damage exhibited by lack of judgment, depression, or limited impulse control while maintaining a high level of intelligence. This deceptive damage hides behind our society's hesitancy to accept prenatal exposure to alcohol as a real problem. We prefer to medicate and call that the cure.

Many FASD victims have others acting as their "seeing eye brain" or "external brain." An adult or more than one adult provides the environment where the FASD brain can succeed to the best of it's ability. This environment is one of structure and constant refocusing, providing the outside brain to compensate for the damaged portions of the FASD brain. This concept was first voiced by Dr. Sterling Clarren, the Robert A. Aldrich Professor of Pediatrics and past Head of the Division of Congenital Defects at the University of Washington School of Medicine in Seattle, Washington.

Understandably, teachers have historically not accepted FASD behaviors in schools. The result leaves an FASD victim, whose behaviors are a result of something they had limited or no control over, looking for acceptance among adults with limited or no success. When that acceptance is not found, the secondary disabilities of FASD take control. Secondary disabilities defined by Dr. Ann Streissguth are, among others, depression, disrupted school experience, trouble with the law, confinement or foster placement, inappropriate sexual behaviors, and mental health problems, drug and alcohol use, and exposure to violence.

A typical middle school, junior high school, or high school

setting with expectations of increased internal controls and increased maturity is not a benign environment for the FASD brain. The FASD brain is emotionally and socially immature, living in a world that expects them to act and think their age.

We don't realize how many times we use shaming and blaming language with children. If truth were to be told, these children would not be able to count, let alone remember, all the times some adult said, "Act your age." Or "How old are you? You sure don't act that age." "What were you thinking?"

'Why don't you remember that?" "I already told you." "What? Do you think I am a dictionary?" These are common unintentional statements by adults responding to behaviors by a brain that can't remember facts, can't think the way you think they should think, can't follow a sequence of directions, forget how to spell, etc. This language drives the FASD brain faster toward outbursts of anger or withdrawing from participating, and ultimately, to the secondary disabilities of depression, trouble in school, and trouble with the law.

I explain adult reaction to behaviors using this analogy: If a blind student walked into my classroom and bumped my water glass off my desk, would I yell, blame, punish, or shame that student? No, I would either place my water glass in another safe location, in other words, accommodate for the student's blindness, or I would teach the student where the water glass would always be. We understand the disability of blindness, so we don't automatically move to the shaming and blaming of the student. Unfortunately, the blind spots in the FASD brain are not physically evident, so the typical adult response to an FASD behavior is shaming and blaming language and punitive responses.

Many times parents are shaming and blaming the victim for behaviors associated with FASD without realizing they are compounding the problem. Many of these children suffer from threats, punishment, and are exposed to abuse up to and including being caged at home, as revealed in nationally reported incidents. Many of the parents are FASD themselves and struggle with parenting skills. The FASD child needs structure to be successful. Many have structure only at school, and that structure may only have punitive responses that do not work for the FASD brain.

These conditions bring on the secondary disabilities of FASD.

101

FASD brain dysfunction leads to depression and brings on alcohol and drug use, a behavior shared by the majority of FASD adolescents. This victim will continue to fall further behind in school and eventually leave the mainstream or completely leave school when forced to take academic courses that are completely outside the realm of possible success. Impulsive actions bring punitive discipline but with little or no resulting change of behavior. In many cases, the illogical male FASD brain reacts violently to the punitive action. This results in more secondary disabilities as defined by Dr. Streissguth, including a disrupted school experience or a record with law enforcement. Anger and frustration are visible signs of the secondary disabilities. With few exceptions, psychologists and psychiatrists will analyze the behaviors of the FASD victim evidenced by the secondary disabilities of depression, anger, and violence and diagnose a mental illness without any acknowledgement or understanding of the real root cause, prenatal exposure to alcohol.

Two sixth grade students were roughhousing while waiting for the bus. As does many times happen, their seemingly harmless antics flared to anger, and quickly erupted into stone throwing. Both boys were from families that were alcohol involved and both had the resulting behaviors of FASD. A rock hit a window, shattering the glass. As their teacher, I was at the scene within seconds and interrupted the action, taking both boys to the office.

Once inside the office, one of the boys quickly agreed he was responsible. The other exploded into violence, smashing anything close. As his temper subsided, both the principal and I explained how both were equally responsible for throwing rocks, even though only one of them threw the rock that hit the window.

I left the office and was walking across the campus, when the boy who thought he was unjustly punished came rushing up to me, his face twisted in anger. I put out my hand to stop him, trying to reason with him and giving him the opportunity to vent his anger toward me. I was completely unprepared for the roundhouse right fist that landed on my left ear. His brain had acted impulsively when throwing rocks, and had been unable or unwilling to accept the consequence, and had acted violently toward me with no thought to the consequence of his action. The only thing that saved me was the fact he was not using something lethal in his attack.

Many people with a normal brain use a fantasy world to cope with reality. Fads such as wannabe gang involvement, Goth, with the influences from nineteenth century Gothic literature and horror movies, Hitler, My Space virtual worlds, manifestos, video games, and fad clothing are mechanisms for the brain to escape from reality or to search for common interests. A normal brain can sort out what is reality and what is fantasy. A normal brain can play a violent video game and understand the fantasy. A normal brain can get deeply involved in Goth or video games without the fantasy becoming reality. An FASD brain, with diminished executive functions, does not have the same capability. The fantasy becomes interwoven into their reality.

All adolescents are influenced by their peers. Group behaviors are well documented and mob mentality is shown on television quite frequently. The FASD brain is influenced in ways a normal brain can resist. Many times, I have witnessed FASD adolescents being goaded into violent behaviors by their peers who knew they could get their dirty work done by these students. Among our staff, we would refer to some of our students as the "bazooka." Other kids would point the "bazooka" at someone they wanted to harm and pull the trigger by convincing them of the need to fight. The "bazooka" would go off with violent results. Many FASD brains live for the adrenalin rush of action, for the acceptance of peers, and the excitement of the fight. When the FASD brain starts to fixate on the solution and begins telling others of his plan, his closest friends, most likely with some of the same brain characteristics, thrive on encouraging him to engage in the violent behaviors, a factor that is hard for the FASD brain to overcome.

And lastly, the whirlwind of factors becomes a "Perfect Storm" when the FASD victim gains access to the fatal weapon. I have seen the appeal weapons have had for students. I have heard stories of the guns on the streets from our students. I saw many drawing of guns and violence. I have seen ammunition brought to school and used in a threatening manner. In the cases of the potential school shooters I dealt with, I know they did not have access to a real gun. If they did, I have no doubt at least one of them would have become one of Minnesota's school shooters, a victim of the "Perfect Storm."

CHAPTER Eight
The Media and the Professionals Do Not Get It
They Are Not Asking the Right Question

Following the Columbine tragedy, President Bush ordered a Secret Services report on school shooters. The sources of the information were court records, investigative reports, school records, and mental health records. Additionally, 10 shooters were interviewed from their jail cells. Unfortunately, this report did not look any further than the behaviors of the perpetrators. The resulting report identified many factors contributing to the spate of school shooters, but did not develop a link between the shooters other than they all were boys.

In the cases of violent incidents, courts, news reporters, law enforcement, public attorneys, social workers, psychologists, psychiatrists, and other mental health professionals are not asking the right questions. These professions are all reactive in nature by trade. They are trained to diagnose a behavior and prescribe a remedy to that behavior, whether it be punitive, medical, or behavioral intervention.

Professionals investigating school shooters are not educators. They are psychologist and sociologists who work in offices or in ivory towers and do not live or work in the trenches. They assume and predict without having the experience of everyday exposure to the kids in question. The investigators did not know they were not asking the most important question.

I sometimes feel like I am cursed with what I know. Every face, every behavior, every parent has to endure the scrutiny of the filters in my brain, filters refined by years of study and experience with brain damage at levels very few have realized or experienced. Other times I feel like an astronomer who looks into deep space for clues of the existence of a star or a galaxy. One can't actually see the actual physical forms, but one can see the clues showing the evidence of the solar mass. One clue links to another, then another, and soon, the clues become the evidence used to determine the existence of the cosmic giant. In the same manner, I look for the researched-based clues that reveal the blind spots in the brain, clues such as academic struggles, deviant social behaviors, disrupted school experience, and prescribed psychotropic medications. I also look for the research-based high-risk factors that indicate a high probability of the mother drinking during pregnancy, clues such as the child being adopted, the drinking habits of the biological mother, where she attended church (some churches do not condemn moderate drinking, others condemn any drinking), where she worked, her age when pregnant, her marriage status when pregnant, did she smoke, and if there was a traumatic event during the pregnancy. Like the astronomer linking clues to make discoveries, I link the clues together to make determinations of the probability of prenatal exposure to alcohol.

Here is your opportunity to link clues. The following article was aired and published by CNN as an anniversary documentary of the Virginia Tech campus shooting. This is an example of all the clues flying in the face of the parents and professionals and their not being able to see the obvious. I am providing this as an exercise in identifying the "red flags" of prenatal exposure to alcohol. All the clues are highlighted in bold. Also, the statements showing the misdiagnosis and the lack of understanding by professionals and the parents of the stark reality of brain damage are highlighted in bold and italics.

"Mom saw warning signs in son who planned shooting spree"

It was just 2½ years ago when Elaine Sonnen found out that her 16-year-old son, Richard, had been planning a Columbine-style attack at his high school.

It would be a fitting payback to his high school classmates who Richard said relentlessly bullied him. "I always wanted to get back at them," Sonnen said of his classmates. "I always wanted to strangle them. ...**I was always mad. I was always angry** and I would come home and cry to mom and dad." Both Richard and Elaine Sonnen spoke to CNN at the 45-acre family farm.

Unlike Columbine and recent school shootings at Northern Illinois University and Virginia Tech, Elaine Sonnen did see the warning signs in her son and was able to stop him. Elaine and her husband, Tom, **adopted Richard from a Bulgarian orphanage** when he was just 4½ years old. "I mean, we just loved him, and he was just a big sparkle of life," she said.

But **only a few months after they brought him home they began to see another side of their son. He was angry and unpredictable**. Elaine Sonnen says at age 6, **Richard told her he wanted to kill her**. She said **he would shake with anger to the point that he'd scream at her, telling her he wanted to destroy her**. "People thought he was just the greatest kid in the world. Very polite, well-mannered, caring," Elaine Sonnen remembered. "At home, **he could be anywhere from just a really helpful kid to a monster. A terrifying monster**." In junior high, he said "evil" classmates started picking on him. Boys and girls, he said, bullied him until he couldn't take it anymore. "I always wanted to get revenge," he told CNN. By the eighth grade, Richard was put on **anti-psychotic medications**. He had been **diagnosed as bipolar and was suffering from obsessive-compulsive disorder and other disorders**. In 1999, when the Columbine shootings happened, the Sonnens feared Richard might do the same thing one day. "We stopped and looked at each other and said, 'This could be Richard, some day this could be him,' " Elaine Sonnen said.

Years later, during his junior year in high school, it turns out they were right. Fed up with the bullies, Richard says he felt like an outcast and started looking for a way to get even. Secretly, he began reading books about Columbine in his school library. The shooters, Eric Harris and Dylan Klebold, became his heroes. "They planned it out so perfectly and so meticulously ... that I just wow, you know," he said. "They're my Gods." He even created his own hit list of the classmates he planned to kill at Prairie High School in Cottonwood, Idaho. "My plan was to set bombs around the school. ... I analyzed a lot of where everybody sat and where everybody did their thing," he said. "I had pinpoints of where I wanted to go, where I wanted to do it."

Harvard Medical School psychologist William Pollack, who consulted on a 2002 federal government study of school shootings, said they found most school shooters often had feelings of anger, sadness and isolation as well as homicidal and suicidal thoughts.

"We see a young man who obviously is telling us how depressed he was, how angry he was and how much he looked up to people who we know are very disturbed and very dangerous and how close he came to killing people," said Pollack, who watched CNN's interview with Richard.

Elaine Sonnen found out about her son's plan during a conversation with him. She ordered him to write down the names of the eight students he wanted dead and then gave the list to his caseworker the next day. Later, he added a teacher and his mother and sister to the hit list. She took immediate action and had her son committed to an Idaho mental institution. Over the next 16 months, he received treatment at several mental health facilities throughout Idaho. "There, I opened up. I felt better. I moved on with myself," Richard said. *"They felt at that point ... they had done everything they could do for him," added Elaine Sonnen. "He was doing great. He could make it on his own. They had no question."*

In January 2007, after almost a year and a half in mental institutions, Richard Sonnen started a new life at Lewis-Clark State College in Lewiston, Idaho. **He was taking a cocktail of three anti-psychotic drugs to help him function**. "[For] the first time in 12 years I was able to hold my son," said Elaine Sonnen. *"So I knew he was on the road to be well."*

Everything seemed to be looking up, but in April of 2007, three days after the Virginia Tech massacre, Richard's mother received a call from police. They told her Richard had made about four different threats to carry out shootings at Lewis-Clark State College and Lewiston High School. Police told her Richard planned to go home, get some guns and go back to school to pull off a sniper attack from a clock tower on the college campus, she told CNN. Police took him into protective custody and searched his apartment for clues. But, in the end, he was released because, authorities say, they didn't have enough evidence to charge him with a crime.

Richard said the whole incident was a big misunderstanding. He said he was telling people about his high school plot and never threatened his college or local high school. But his mother doesn't believe his version of the story. "No. I believe he made those threats," she said. "I still believe it."

Richard, now 19, signed an order banning him from campus for one year. Today, he lives on his own in the state of Washington. He's still on medication but not seeing a psychiatrist. Since he's over the age of 18 his mom can't force him to go.

Is Elaine Sonnen still afraid of her son? "Yeah, at times, I'm very afraid," she said. "Because he still has a lot of anger towards me." She said the **signs are still there and she fears what could happen if he ever stops taking his medicine**. "He's not getting the help and the insight from a professional that could see the signs," she said. *"Because, as a person with a mental illness, you have skewed thinking."* Even though Richard calls her the "greatest person in the world," Elaine Sonnen still protects the family by keeping an alarm on her son's bedroom door when he comes home to visit.

So why are Richard Sonnen and his mother, Elaine, speaking out now? In the wake of the Northern Illinois University and Virginia Tech shootings, Richard wants young people experiencing the same symptoms he had to seek out help. His mother wants parents and authorities to listen for warning signs and to act fast and decisively.

I used this real media story word for word to highlight exactly what I have been telling you in the prior chapters. Did you find the same thing I found? Now that you know the exhibitions of brain damage from prenatal exposure and the risk factors of biological mothers drinking during pregnancy, you can see this young man exhibits brain damage from prenatal exposure to alcohol. I would suggest to his adoptive mother to read the research on Fetal Alcohol Spectrum Disorders, so she will understand why she has not been able to hold her son. After she fully comprehends the brain damage sustained when her son's biological mother prenatally exposed him to alcohol, she will understands statements such as *"So I knew he was on the road to be well"* are, unfortunately, unrealistic. She will then know her son will always need someone to be his "Seeing Eye Brain." She will realize her son is at risk to act in a violent manner at any time and will most likely not be emancipated from adult care until the age of thirty-five or older. Chances are, either she or a social agency will have to be the structure to assist his adult brain, and if not, the judicial system will take over when he acts on his violent thought patterns. He may get better, but he will never be well.

Here is another example of actions that are so horrific you ask yourself, "How could someone do something like that?" Or "Why would someone do something like that?" When I read news accounts of violent acts, the same questions go through my mind and I look for the clues that will give me some indication whether the actions were a result of something unspoken. In this story, the truth is buried using a couple of words, words on a page only understood by someone who knows that they truly mean.

"Father asks judge to accept plea, avoid trial"
Dave Kolpack , *Star Tribune*

FARGO, N.D. - The father of a Wisconsin teenager accused of killing his sister in Fargo has written a letter to the judge in the case, asking him to reconsider a plea agreement and spare his family a trial.

"It's my beautiful daughter that has been murdered by my son," the Rev. Scott Carlson wrote in a letter to Judge John Irby. "I have heard his confession. I know what he did. I know the horror of my daughter's last moments on this earth. That is an image that will remain with me for a long time."

Sergei Carlson, 16, is charged with murder and a deviant sexual act in the death of his 16-year-old sister, Whitney Carlson. Irby rejected a plea agreement in May that called for a sentence of 30 years in prison.

In his letter to Irby, Rev. Carlson, of Sun Prairie Wisconsin, said the judge's rejection of the plea deal made him feel as if he had been kicked in the stomach.

"I'm asking you to please reconsider this judgment," Carlson wrote.

Carlson told The Associated Press on Thursday that he decided to make the letter public because he had not heard from the judge. Defense attorney Mark Beauchene declined comment. Rod Olson, the Cass County court administrator, said Judge Irby did not feel it would be appropriate to discuss the letter.

Prosecutors would not talk about the specifics of the letter.

"We're mindful of Sergei Carlson's right to a fair trial. We want to make sure that we preserve that right," said Reid Brady, Cass County prosecutor. "We don't fault the father, either. We wouldn't criticize him at all. At the same time, we respect the judge's decision."

Authorities said Sergei Carlson told police he strangled his sister in her bedroom with his hands, put pillows over her face to muffle her sounds, then had sexual contact with her.

The two-page letter from Scott Carlson, dated June 1, was included in the case file but sealed from public view. Carlson faxed it to media outlets Thursday, along with a cover letter explaining his frustration with the judge's ruling.

"The sad news is that because of his decisions, not only does our family continue to endure a lengthy process that could have and should have been done a month ago," Carlson said. "But as we move closer and closer to a trial, the reality is this will continue for a long time."

Carlson said he is upset that more details of the crime will become public during a trial that will "come at a great cost" to the taxpayers of North Dakota.

Beauchene said in court documents that Irby would only accept a sentence of life in prison with the possibility of parole. Beauchene said that showed bias toward his client and he asked for a new judge. Irby refused the request, but ordered the trial moved from Fargo.

Have you found the words? There certainly are "red flags" of brain damage in the article up to this point, those being **strangled his sister in her bedroom with his hands**, and **then had sexual contact with her**. These are violent, illogical, horrible acts by a 16-year old, acts that are not that of a normal brain. But these red flags are not the main clue. The article continues:

Sergei Carlson, called Isaac by family members, was adopted from Russia when he was 7 years old and moved with his father to Wisconsin in 2002. Whitney Carlson lived with her mother in Fargo. Sergei, Whitney and three other sisters alternated between parents for summers and holidays.

Scott Carlson concluded the letter to Irby by telling the judge how difficult it has been to explain these new details of the case to his daughters.

"Words cannot express the depth and pain and grief I feel in the death of my daughter, Whitney. I miss her greatly," Carlson wrote. "But I also know how much I have invested in Isaac, through adopting him and welcoming him into our family. I know the energy I have put in to give him a shot at a life.

"While I certainly want to have him held accountable for what he has done, I also want to give him a shot at rehabilitation and a life," Scott Carlson wrote. "That is why I felt this plea agreement was a good one."

Did you find the words? This boy **was adopted from Russia**. Children adopted from Russian are at an extremely high risk for prenatal exposure to alcohol. Do I know for certain he was prenatally exposed? No. Do I know for certain his actions are exhibitions of a brain damaged by prenatal exposure to alcohol? Yes. Here is a brain damaged to the point of being incapable of controlling the sexual impulses raging through his body, impulses that drove him to murder and unspeakable sexual deviancy. The media needs to ask the right questions, to ask the "why", and to not stop asking until they find the cause rooted in the damaged brains of our violent and deviant offenders. Then clearly and unequivocally to report the link between the drinking of the mothers and the behaviors of the offenders.

Two States - Seven School Shooters – All Fit the Profile

T hroughout my years as a school administrator I have been keenly aware of the dangerous situations other principals and teachers have experienced in school shooting incidents. Every school shooting brought back memories of a little know tragedy in my hometown. When the Red Lake, MN shooting occurred in 2005, I started to see a link not seen by anyone else. My educational experience on Minnesota reservations, along with my memories of my hometown's school shooting, placed me in a unique position to see this connection. Seeing the link was the easy part. Confirming it was the difficult part.

A news report showing the fourth grade picture of the Red Lake shooter, Jeff Weise, was the catalyst for my research. Years of working with prenatally exposed children living on or near reservations across Minnesota gave me the ability to immediately see the physical clues of prenatal exposure to alcohol. News articles confirmed his mother's heavy drinking. As I had with all the shooters before him, I compared him with what I knew about the shooter in my hometown in 1966. For the first time, I started to wonder if the Grand Rapids' shooter had the same characteristics as Jeff Weise, Minnesota's third and most prolific school shooter.

Preliminary research of the Grand Rapids shooting seemed to fit my theory. People familiar with the long ago happenings seemed to remember facts that supported a link of prenatal exposure to alcohol. As I looked into this link and began to write about my findings, I realized a much more detailed search for facts was warranted and the journey toward writing this book began.

I started with the intent of comparing the Grand Rapids, MN shooting of 1966 and the Red Lake shooting of 2005. The Rocori Cold Springs, MN shooting of 2003 was a natural addition to the study. Shortly after I started, Eric Hainstock became the third shooter from Wisconsin. He seemed to fit the profile I was beginning to form. As I looked into the details of that tragedy, I found information on a 1969 school shooting in Tomah, WI. which was consistent with others I was documenting. I decided to include the three school shooters from Wisconsin in my search for a common root cause. Eventually, I added a seventh shooter who was born and raised in Minnesota prior to moving to Arkansas with his mother, where he committed a shocking school shooting, becoming one of the two youngest children in our nation charged with murder.

Gathering information on shooters from years ago was difficult, due to the factors of time, lost memories, an entirely different view of juvenile crime, and the reticence of some to bring back memories of the tragedy. To gather the most accurate information possible on the shootings that happened over twenty years ago, I traveled to the locations and had personal conversations with the law enforcement officers and others involved. The research was both difficult and rewarding. Some people involved still recall with amazing detail what they went through on the day of the shooting. Others have chosen to forget. Finding information on the mother of the shooter was much more difficult than finding details on the shooter, the shooter's father, the victims, and the events. Eye witness confirmations of her drinking patterns by more than one person or by family members were required before I would make a positive determination the mother drank while pregnant. The people who provided the information and confirmation are not revealed, as this study brought me in contact with many people who were willing to tell me the information, but not willing to have their participation made public.

I asked people to describe the behaviors of the shooter in school, at home, and in the community. I asked people to describe the drinking habits of the mother, if any. I asked for the church affiliation of the mother, if any. I looked at the news reports to find identifying behavioral, academic, and physical characteristics of the shooter. I read every blog or forum I could find that discussed any of the Minnesota or Wisconsin school shootings. I asked questions on blogs and websites. I found information in libraries, historical societies, and newspapers. I talked to local people in bars, in restaurants, and at local businesses. I followed leads without revealing who provided me with the information. Any information gained was checked and rechecked.

Much more information was readily available in the later shooting cases. I was able to confirm alcoholic patterns of the mothers in two cases using news reports. In both cases, no connection was made by any reporter or commentator between the behaviors of the shooter and the drinking habits of the mother.

What I found is irrefutable. Every school shooter in Minnesota and Wisconsin fits the profile of prenatal exposure to alcohol. **In every case, the behaviors of the shooter fit research-based social and academic exhibitions of brain damage. In four cases, heavy prenatal exposure to alcohol is absolutely confirmed.** In one of the remaining two cases, while the shooter fits the profile of prenatal exposure, the mother denies drinking while pregnant. In the remaining case, although the academic and social behaviors, as well as secondary disabilities of depression, alcohol use, and a disrupted school experience, fit the profile of prenatal exposure to alcohol, no information has been found to either confirm or deny prenatal alcohol exposure.

Furthermore, another school shooter was born and raised in Minnesota prior to moving to Jonesboro, Arkansas. In the case of this seventh shooter linked to Minnesota/Wisconsin study, **he fits the profile of prenatal exposure to alcohol. His confirmed mother's binge drinking patterns at that time of her life, puts him at a**

very high probability of prenatal exposure to alcohol.

Each of the seven school shooters are examined in this chapter. Each event is examined for the red flags of prenatal exposure to alcohol. Two of the following school shootings were committed in the 1960's and are not a part of the nation's conscience. I bring you these stories not to glorify the tragedy, but to bring to focus the fact that adolescent boys with brain damage were committing horrific crimes before Goth, violent television and movies, and violent video games. Each mother's history of behaviors is examined in as much detail as I could locate. Findings that either confirmed the mother prenatally exposing the child or that would place her at high risk for prenatally exposing her son to alcohol are presented for each mother. The facts reveal, for the first time, the untold truth.

The investigation and writing of each story is a story onto itself, something I will strive to tell without taking away from the message. I chose to place the Minnesota and Wisconsin school shootings in chronological order, starting with the first fatal school shooting by an adolescent in the United States that I could find. It happened in my hometown.

Grand Rapids, MN

October 5, 1966, Mrs. Hanson, one of the three school nurses in Grand Rapids, Minnesota, drove into her parking place at the southeast parking lot. She thought she was late, as there did not seem to be anyone in the common area between the glassed-in entrance of the high school and the large gymnasium. This area was usually bustling with students visiting with each other before the start of the school day. Her view of this area was partially blocked by the district administration building.

Her son, a senior, had ridden in with her from the small community of Warba rather than ride the school bus. As the two of them hurried toward the entrance, a short, dark haired David Black burst around the corner of the administration building holding a big black pistol pointed in front of him. He had a strange blank-eyed look on his face. Mrs. Hanson recalled thinking he was bringing a gun to school to show his teachers and purposely did not make eye contact with him. Guns were not common, but not unheard of, since Grand Rapids High School had a target practice room where students and community members could bring their guns for practice.

Mrs. Hanson and her son continued into the school, walking through a strangely silent group of students. Since she thought maybe she was late, she passed through the silent students without inquiring about their odd behavior. She went to her office and only then did she find out she had just come face to face with the first school shooter in Minnesota and quite possibly in the nation. Mrs. Hanson had just had a brush with death.

David Black, the Grand Rapids shooter, was never a friendly person. His father was emotionally and physically abusive. His mother was emotionally abusive to the point of seeming to not want him around. His parents married young, with his mother being sixteen years old at the time. His father traveled and ruled with an iron fist when he was home. His mother let him do whatever he wanted and did not have any disciplinary control over him. She would tell him he was stupid in front of others. He did not make friends easily and was never likable, according to someone who grew up with him.

My search for evidence of David Black's behaviors resulted in a phone call to a relative of his who was also his classmate. At the beginning of the phone conversation, she had told me David's mother did not drink any alcohol. She described all she could remember of David's behaviors she had observed in and out of school. She was the same age as David and was in classes with him. I listened to her describe behaviors of a prenatally exposed boy. As she described his behaviors and his family life, I kept asking if it were possible his mother had a couple of binges or was a closet alcoholic. Again and again, she expressed confidence in her memory of his mother. The phone conversation concluded with her saying she would talk to her mother, who knew David's mother intimately, to find out if her memory of David's mother was correct. If I heard from her again, she would have new information. If I did not hear from her, what she said was the truth.

I could hardly sleep that night. All the behavioral information she provided placed David Black at a very high probability of brain damage from prenatal exposure to alcohol. How could I be wrong?

I began doubting my ability to identify the red flags of prenatal exposure to alcohol to the point of being physically sick. If David Black fit the profile but was not prenatally exposed, I was wrong in my belief that prenatal exposure to alcohol was the root cause for school shooting behaviors.

The next morning an email was waiting for me. "I stand corrected - Leora Black drank a lot and her first baby died." She went on to say David Black's mother continued to drink through her other two pregnancies. I immediately expressed my gratefulness to my source for her willingness to follow through and find the truth. David Black was heavily prenatally exposed to alcohol. The fatal link was undeniable.

David Black had, what one classmate called, "an active storybook mind," someone who always told stories to impress his friends, stories that were outside the realm of possibility. He had been teased since elementary school. In junior high science class one day when the teacher walked out of the room, one of his tormentors told him if he drank some formaldehyde, he could be part of their group. He drank the required dose and became the laughing stock of the class once again. He got into trouble and the tormentors did not. As he grew older, he was the subject of ridicule because he was short and wide and heavily whiskered. It was said he should have shaved twice a day. He told the only friend he seemed to have, Mark Lebeck, that he was a tough guy with mafia connections, that he had a pilot's license and he had an alcohol making still out in the woods. Lebeck told others, and the others, who were older, laughed it off and told Lebeck that Black was lying. Lebeck told Black what the older students were saying and Black was feeling the brunt of their ridicule.

He was considered different, someone who was a little strange. He was not a good student, but was not held to high expectations either. He had a history of disciplinary actions throughout his school years. This was an era before special education, so there were no disability designations, no special education assessments, no special education classes, and no special considerations for disabilities. He was making his way through school as best he could, without the supports that a student with his disabilities would have in our current system.

David's demeanor and behaviors brought ridicule. He had tried to make the football team, but had been cut. His clothing was not new, he did not take good care of his hygiene. He was from the west end of town, from the poor side of town. He was used as a verbal punching bag by his so-called friends. They assumed he liked being teased, since he kept coming back for more. They did not know that his damaged brain, made so by his mother's drinking, made a decision to teach his tormentors a lesson. He brought bullets to school and told his main tormentor he was going to kill him the next day, which drew the same response as his other tall tales.

That night, he asked his dad to teach him how to load the .22 pistol he knew his father had. His dad brought out the gun and showed him how to load it. In the morning, his buddies were waiting in their typical spot after smoking their morning cigarettes, totally unaware of his intent. To their surprise and shock, he came across the parking lot flashing a pistol and pointed it at the group, becoming the tough guy as he had threatened. The group scattered, leaving an older high school student, Kevin Roth, rooted to the spot. Black fired one shot, hitting Roth in the chest, collapsing his lung and missing his heart by a fraction of an inch. Roth crouched and ran over to a teacher, crying out, "Help me, help me. He shot me." The teacher, not hearing any shot and thinking he was messing around, said, "Why don't you grow up." Roth made his way into the hallway where he collapsed. Another teacher nudged him with his shoe and told him to get up.

Meanwhile, Mark Lebeck, one of the fleeing students, told Forrest Willey, an administrator in the building, what was happening. Upon hearing there was a shooter in the school yard, Willey immediately exclaimed, "We need to protect the students and others and get that gun away from him." He swiftly confronted Black, who fired one shot but missed his target. Mr. Willey demanded the gun. Black fired two more shots at Mr. Willey and hit him in the stomach. As Black stood near his fallen victim, the football coach, Noble Hall, without thinking of his own safety, rushed up to Mr. Willey. He picked him up, and carried him out of the line of fire. After watching this heroic action within a couple of feet from the barrel of his still loaded pistol, Black turned and ran around the corner of the administration building, where he rushed past Mrs. Hanson. Mrs. Hanson has often thought if she had challenged David

121

Black, he would have shot her like he shot and killed Forrest L. Willey.

Black continued across the street and hunkered down behind a tree firing his last two bullets at the first police officer who arrived on the scene. Harvey Dahline, a young part-time uniformed police officer, part-time bus driver, happened to be driving toward the school when he was intercepted by a Minnesota State Trooper. Dahline drove his loaded bus into a protected parking lot and jumped into action. He borrowed a pistol from the trooper and moved toward the scene. After a quick conference with a police officer who was pinned down by Black's fire, he sprinted to a tree close to Black. By this time, Black stood in the open school yard, surrounded by a semi-circle of curious and shocked students. Dahline approached Black with his gun pointed to the ground, not wanting to shoot because of the number of students who were watching the horrifying scene. After about 5 minutes, he convinced Black to drop his gun. Black dropped the gun and as Black moved toward him, Officer Dahline saw he was holding his right hand in a peculiar position. Dahline demanded Black open his hand. A knife dropped to the ground. Black later told Dahline he was going to stab him when he got close enough. Black appeared dazed and bewildered as Dahline apprehended him.

Back at the shooting scene, Kevin Roth's injury was deemed more critical than Mr. Willey's. Both were quickly taken to the hospital, but eight days later Mr. Willey died, leaving a grieving family and community.

"Seldom, if ever, has an educator demonstrated so unselfishly his complete dedication to the welfare of his students as did Forrest Willey," the Grand Rapids School District said in a resolution adopted on the day of his funeral. "With no concern for his personal safety, he risked and gave up his own life to prevent the serious injury and possible death of young people in our district."

Grand Rapids quickly seemed to move back to normal for everyone except the families of the victims. Black received a 25-year murder sentence and a concurrent 10-year sentence for aggravated assault on the student. After five years in the state prison, he was put on a work release program. He was paroled when he reached the age of 21.

Within a short time after his release, he was arrested for

molesting a young boy while working in a hobby shop. When the police investigated the molestation, they uncovered another one a few days earlier. He pled guilty to second-degree criminal sexual conduct and served another four years in prison. He never returned to live in Grand Rapids, moving to another state where he worked at menial custodial jobs.

Mark Lebeck, the one friend of David Black, committed suicide a few years following the shooting. There is no evidence as to why he committed suicide.

David Black's mother and father were alcoholics. His mother hit and killed a man while driving a car when pregnant with her first child, an event that drove her deeper into the bottle. She drank so heavily she lost her first child. She continued drinking through her second and third pregnancies, in which she bore her son David and a daughter. Her alcoholic behaviors exposed David to heavy amounts of alcohol in utero. David Black clearly fits the profile of a 15 year old heavily impacted by prenatal exposure to alcohol. His behaviors, his academic struggles, his fantasy world, telling big falsehoods, his illogical attempted murder of Roth and impulsive murder of Forrest Wiley are all exhibited behaviors of brain damage. The fact that his mother prenatally exposed him to alcohol confirms the evidence of his brain damage. His brain experienced the "Perfect Storm" of mitigating factors.

As I delved deeper into the background of David Black's mother, a phone call brought an entirely new perspective to my investigation of the shooting. I was talking to Harvey Dahline, a now retired Grand Rapids police officer who had arrested David Black. Early in the call, after I explained why I was researching school shooters, he said, "You are going to think I am crazy." When I heard those words, my response was, "Try me."

I had approached my interview with him with memories of this strong police officer who had built a reputation of fairness in my hometown. He continued by saying, "I have what you are talking about. My mother was a heavy drinker. She drank while she was pregnant with me. I was taken from her when I was six years old. I have always had trouble with things, but I have worked hard to overcome them."

This now older man did not hide anything. He told of the hard upbringing in central and northern Minnesota, moving from foster family to orphanage, and back to foster homes. He spoke of poor schooling and of being ridiculed for his poor reading and writing skills. He spoke of being punished when he did not get good marks on his school work. He never received one-on-one help at school. He showed me his report cards that showed poor marks for everything, including how he sat in his chair. He did not have good memories of his early school years and explained he only had a ninth grade education.

How could someone such as Harvey, with prenatal exposure to alcohol, have such a different outcome from the shooters detailed in this book? That fateful day in October, one prenatally exposed fifteen-year-old was standing in the schoolyard with a gun and a knife. He was confronted and arrested by another prenatally exposed young man. What a contrast! What made the difference?

Dahline was an athlete, a status none of the school shooters attained. The prenatal exposure had damaged his ability to learn to some extent, but he was a physical specimen. His physical appearance did not create an atmosphere of ridicule from his peers. Even though he had plenty of shaming and blaming heaped on him by adults for his limited academic ability, he was recognized by his peers as someone who was above average when it came to physical ability. In fact, during the first week of high school football practice, his coach, Noble Hall, the hero who later carried Forrest Willey out of the line of fire, told Dahline to take it easy on his teammates at practice because he was hitting them so hard on every play.

Dahline took advantage of his physical abilities, working in jobs that minimized his deficiencies. Dahline entered the National Guard at age sixteen. There, he was in a highly structured environment with an opportunity to learn skills that helped him in his career. He displayed a determination to overcome his deficiencies. He freely speaks of those deficiencies, his struggles to write and to remember names, among them.

He proudly served our country in Korea. Upon coming home, he worked in several jobs and married. His wife became his "Seeing Eye Brain" when he needed the help. She found a little ad in the paper calling for candidates to take the civil service test needed to become a police officer in the city of Grand Rapids. He did not think he could pass the test. She thought he could. He recalled the strategy he used to take the test, only answering the ones he knew, then going back over the others and answering with his best guess. He had the highest score and became a police officer, entering a profession that gave him a life of structure and accountability and made use of his physical abilities. He had mastered strategies that compensated for his deficiencies. He was in a job where he could use his assets, rather than be frustrated by his disabilities. He didn't drink alcohol. He did not want to end up like his mother.

When visiting with him and his wife, they both commented on reading my manuscript and having a better understanding of what they had experienced in their lives together. When I mentioned the other adult being the "seeing eye brain," his wife clearly understood that had been her role throughout their marriage.

I was struck by their openness and commitment to helping get this story out. Because of his struggles in his early life, I believe Harvey Dahline, without realizing why, had a better understanding of David Black than anyone else at the scene at that exact moment in time when he walked out into the line of fire toward him. I also believe, after talking to him about his life and remembering him as I do, his self-professed prenatal exposure to alcohol deficiencies were turned into gifts that he used as a long-standing, highly respected public servant for the citizens of Grand Rapids, MN.

Tomah, WI

Three years after the Grand Rapids shooting, in late November, 1969, the Tomah School Board in Tomah, Wisconsin, was wrestling with decisions like: "How long should the female student's skirts be? Should they be four inches above the knee or should we allow the girls to wear slacks?" In one terrifying series of shotgun blasts, Tomah changed forever.

I would not have known there was a school shooting in Tomah, WI, if my Google search had not found The Mogensen Lecture Series, which is part of a collaborative leadership in education outreach effort established to honor Martin Mogensen, a 1952 University of Wisconsin-Eau Claire graduate. The story behind the lecture series included the reason Martin Mogensen was being honored. A student had killed him in his school office in 1969. His daughters, Marti Mogensen and Margaret Mogensen Nelson Brinkhaus, both graduates of UW-Eau Claire, and other family members and friends were instrumental in keeping his legacy alive through the Martin Mogensen Education Lecture Fund of the UW-Eau Claire Foundation.

I could find very little about the Tomah shooting beyond the articles about the lecture series. I knew I had to visit the town and try to find information in the library or historical society or by sitting in the bars and restaurants, asking people if they knew anything about the shooter.

Finding the truth forty years after the fact is not easy. My initial contacts gave me the name of the shooter, but did not want to talk about him. They connected me with others who did talk, but I had to analyze the relationships of the source to the shooter, and decide if the information was valid. People close to the shooter's family were most likely going to paint as good a picture as possible of the mother and family. Others want the truth to be told and are willing to break down the wall of silence around the mother. I needed to find the individuals who had first hand knowledge of the mother and were willing to tell the story without prejudice.

The nearly 40 year old news reports of the shooting and court actions reflected the times, with the shooter being tried as a juvenile with no mention of the name of the shooter. Only through the help of people near to the tragedy could the truth about the mother's drinking patterns come out. After several calls, I had narrowed the search and was able to find someone who had first hand information and was willing to tell the story.

The school shooter was a fourteen year old by the name of Richard "Dickie" Anderson. He lived in a troubled family. His father could not hold a job and was away from home a lot. The school social worker had been involved because of Dickie's problems and reported a lack of follow-through by both his mother and father. Dickie had been living with his grandmother due to problems at home.

News reports stated Anderson had "school phobia" and did not want to go to school. He had been getting into trouble with the principal, Mr. Mogensen, for at least two years, showing "anti-social" behaviors. In fact, he was missing so much school, the school was recommending psychological testing. Twice, when asked to take their son to the scheduled testing, the parents did not respond. The school social worker had determined the family situation was not healthy. On the morning of the shooting, Mr. Mogensen called Anderson's mother to tell her he was truant and of his plans to have a judge order a psychological assessment of Dickie Anderson. Reportedly, Anderson's mother confronted her son on the day of the shooting. Anderson, realizing he was at the point of possibly getting sent away, stated at his court hearing he "had the impulse to kill Mogensen." According to his doctor's testimony at the trial, the thought seemed logical to Anderson and he couldn't stop himself.

Shortly after 12:30, November 19, 1969, this troubled fourteen year old student walked into the principal's office and fired a shot at Principal Martin Mogensen, who was talking on the phone. Mogensen was hit on the elbow and managed to escape to his private office, but before he could protect himself, Anderson fired more shots, a total of five, hitting him in the back and killing the father of six children.

Anderson walked past the horrified secretary and a female student who had watched the tragic events take place in front of them. He stood in the hall holding the gun until police arrived. A teacher, Mr. Thies, approached the boy in the hall. Anderson demanded to see the Undersheriff, Ray Harris, who, tragically, was home grieving after finding out that same day about the loss of his younger brother in Vietnam. Anderson knew Harris because the officer had questioned him two weeks earlier. The fourteen year old had been accused of the random, senseless killing of a cow. Thies moved to safety when he realized Anderson was not going to drop the gun.

Harris was called to the scene and approached Anderson, who stood in the hallway with one live shell in the pump action 20 gauge. Harris was afraid he was going to be targeted because of the cow incident. He was also afraid for his kindergarten daughter, now safely locked in a classroom in the basement. He slowly moved down the hallway toward Anderson, ready to hit the floor if Anderson made an aggressive move with the gun. As he got close,

Anderson dropped the gun.

Anderson had a history of problems. His parents reported he "had manifested repressed aggression and hostility" since the age of four. He had used anti-social behaviors to call attention to himself. He displayed anxiety and depression. He had been in many fights with other students and had physical altercations with teachers. He smoked and admitted taking LSD and pep pills. He had great difficulty attending school. He did not like to take instructions or orders from adults.

Anderson attended school prior to testing for Special Education and before many of the current behavioral diagnosis had been "discovered." According to news reports, his school phobia began when he was twelve years old, when the typical prenatally exposed brain hits a plateau for math and reading. The usual upper elementary curriculum requires the brain to think in the abstract. A damaged brain has great difficulty moving from the concrete to the abstract. If there are no adaptations or an understanding of the difficulty, the student uses the avoidance strategies of skipping, outbursts, and anti-social behaviors. His pattern of behaviors is classic FASD.

For the first time, the truth is to be told in the Tomah shooting case. A person with intimate knowledge of the Anderson family revealed Dickie Anderson's father, Bob, was a heavy alcoholic. Dickie Anderson's mother was pregnant when she married Dickie's dad. She was drunk at the wedding, revealing the fact that she did not change her drinking habits when pregnant. Anderson's mother was at the bars drinking with his dad whenever they went out. The parents did a lot of drinking and fighting. Both parents continued to drink throughout their lives, with Bob Anderson dying years later after coming home drunk and taking cough medicine. According to a person very close to the family, Dickie's younger sister was "not smart," which fits the profile of the damage caused by a drinking mother. Since Anderson was born in the 1950's, Mrs. Anderson did not have any idea her drinking habit was damaging her children's brains.

Anderson was a victim of heavy prenatal exposure to alcohol. This does not excuse his behavior. It explains his behavior. The behaviors identified in the news accounts, the cow killing, his parent's descriptions of his behavior, and by witness accounts, as

128

well as the illogical violent murder of the principal are exhibitions of the brain damage from alcohol exposure.

This was the first school shooting in Wisconsin on record, a little over three years after the first school shooting in Minnesota. Like Minnesota, there were no television stations at the scene, no satellite trucks beaming stories around the world. The local newspaper reporter walked into the office and took photos of the shattered windows and walls peppered with shotgun pellets without having to cross any police tape. The local and statewide papers headlined the story but the rest of the nation was unaware of the tragedy. His name was not published locally and, because of his age, he was adjudicated to a juvenile placement in a mental institution. His family left Tomah. He was later known to brag about killing a principal and on at least in two different occasions, came back to Tomah and got into fights. Anderson died in a car accident years later.

School shootings were occurring across the nation throughout the late 1960's, 70's, and 80's. Wisconsin and Minnesota did not experience another school shooting until the early 90's. By then, the shootings in Grand Rapids and Tomah were mostly forgotten outside of the two communities. A 1993 murder in Wauwatosa, Wisconsin, was the first fatal school shooting in the two states in twenty-four years.

Wauwatosa, WI

Wednesday morning, December 1, 1993, Leonard McDowell arrived at his menial job more agitated than usual. He was known to have a quick violent temper and his co-workers steered clear of him this morning. They could tell something was not right. At twenty-one, he was already an alcoholic and this morning, he appeared to have been drinking.

Three years of fermenting hate was about to boil over. McDowell, no stranger to the local law enforcement and school authorities, had chosen this day to drink himself to the point of acting on his hate.

Three years earlier, McDowell had been removed from school for assaulting a teacher. He had grabbed a teacher by the head, kissed her on the cheek, pushed her to the ground, then kissed her on the cheek again. This blatant sexual assault caused him to be arrested and charged with assault. Less than two weeks later, he was arrested for making obscene phone calls. He was suspended for that incident. He came back on school grounds during his suspension and was removed from the school again. Months later, he was arrested for disorderly conduct for refusing to leave the school grounds. The Associate Principal, Dale Breitlow was the person who had held McDowell accountable for his actions.

After McDowell's graduation, he was cited several times for loitering on school property and underage drinking. He was charged with receiving stolen property in connection with a series of apartment robberies. His crimes continued as he was accused of threatening a member of his family. Neighbors had grown accustomed to seeing him being arrested. Unfortunately, his arrests did not lead to a change in his life. According to McDowell, he decided Mr. Breitlow had to die or McDowell himself would have to die. The 21 year-old drop-out walked into the high school in Wauwautosa and shot Assistant Principal Dale Breitlow.

This school shooting did not fit the pattern of the other Minnesota and Wisconsin school shootings because of the age of the shooter. Fourteen and fifteen year olds committed the other school shootings. The media paid little attention to Mc Dowell's parents because he was an adult. His mother refused to talk to news reporters. When I inquired, both the Milwaukee public defender and the Wauwatosa police chief, who was involved in the arrest in 1993, said no one thought to ask if the mother had a drinking habit. This case is one that fits the profile, but no evidence was found of any drinking habits of the mother because of the difficulty of tracing her whereabouts when she was pregnant with McDowell. I did not find any pictures of McDowell when he was young, as physical characteristics are easier to determine at a younger age. I did receive photos taken by the police when he was arrested at age twenty-one. He does display an indistinct philtrum and thin upper lip, both potential indicators of prenatal exposure to alcohol. Clearly alcohol played a part, as he was drunk at the time of the shooting.

The study of the Wauwatosa shooting was particularly difficult due to the peculiar lifestyle of his parents. His parents lived in two other states prior to moving to Wisconsin. Leonard McDowell's father had not been in Leonard's life since he had a sex change when Leonard was very young.

Cold Spring, MN

Another ten years passed before Minnesota or Wisconsin experienced another school shooting. September 24, 2003, dawned like any other fall day in the small Minnesota town of Cold Spring. The trees were beginning to turn to their beautiful fall colors and the football season was in full swing. This scene had played out for generations of families who worked the rock quarry and ran the surrounding businesses and farms.

Fifteen-year-old John Jason McLaughlin went to school that morning with an intent to kill. For reasons known only to him, he decided to become a murderer.

He confronted a classmate, fourteen-year-old Seth Bartell, with his dad's .22-caliber handgun. He had stolen the gun and brought it to school in his backpack. His first shot wounded Seth in the chest. The second shot missed Seth, fatally wounding Aaron Rollins, who was nearby. McLaughlin chased the fleeing Bartell and shot him in the forehead.

A heroic teacher shouted "No" at McLaughlin, when the teen pointed the pistol at him. The loud shout broke McLaughlin's focus on killing. He then emptied the bullets from the gun and dropped it.

Aaron Rollins died that day. Seth Bartell died sixteen days later and was later falsely branded as a bully by McLaughlin's defense attorney.

Studying this case was particularly disturbing. The fact that the shooter's father was a deputy sheriff made finding the truth more difficult. My requests to the county sheriff for information were ignored, which was much different than with other shootings. The editor of the newspaper did not want to provide any information. I was stymied by a wall of silence.

The shooter was characterized as being teased and bullied in an attempt to blame one of the victims. That, and the fact that the perpetrator was the son of a deputy sheriff, put the Bartell family

131

under scrutiny without unconditional support from the law enforcement community. Prior to the trial, Seth's parent's house was secretly searched, with the intruders leaving doors open in their hurry to escape when someone came home. The defense attorney sent investigators to another town where the Bartells had lived, trying to dig up dirt on Seth. The defense did everything they could to vilify Seth Bartell in the press to provide a motive for the killing.

They found nothing, but still stained his legacy in their attempt to blame the victim. Not a single witness at the trial saw or heard anything that would remotely implicate Seth Bartell as an instigator. McLaughlin's love interest, when asked to describe Seth on the witness stand, said one word, "Inspirational." His nonverbal response to her statement in the courtroom was to glare at her with hatred in his eyes. He was found guilty of first and second-degree murder and sentenced to life in prison.

The news reports tended to be kind to McLaughlin and his parents. I could not find one mention of his mother's behaviors. There seemed to be a general sense of bewilderment as to how the son of a law officer could do such a thing. Unfortunately, the entire story was not told at trial. The prosecution presented only what was needed to convict him of murder and nothing more. The public did not hear that he had earlier shot a mailman with a paintball gun.

McLaughlin's father had found out he had been experimenting with bombs and had written about blowing up a drug store when he was in seventh grade. There were public reports stating McLaughlin had a history of discipline issues at school. He had begun to withdraw from his friends over the months prior to the shooting. His mother told the court he was suffering from a mental illness. His friends described him as intensely shy and self-conscious about his acne. He told a friend he was being tested to see if he had a split-personality disorder.

The judge stated in the trial that McLaughlin had "some sort of mental impairment." The prosecutor agreed McLaughlin has some sort of mental illness associated with depression. He had a history of lying and exaggerating to his parents and friends. He was small and short. His nickname was "Shrimp." While awaiting prosecution, McLaughlin was diagnosed with a metal illness and was taking medication.

Classmates of McLaughlin's mother said she drank and enjoyed partying in high school. A highly reputable source who knew her throughout the past 20 years told me she was a "conservative drinker". Mary McLaughlin told me in a telephone call that she did not drink when pregnant with her son, Jason. She was responding to a letter I had sent to her asking her the question. She said she was a drinker in her younger days, but when her brother was seriously injured in an alcohol related car accident, she changed her drinking habits and didn't drink like she had before the accident. The accident happened years before her son was born. She said that she now has an occasional drink. She said the shooting was a result of her son's mental illness and bullying at school, not a result of alcohol or drugs.

John Jason McLaughlin was the second school shooter in Minnesota. Some believe his behaviors were a result of him thinking he could get away with things because his father was a deputy sheriff. This case represents the dilemma of my study. McLaughlin's behaviors, his diagnosed mental illness, prescribed medication, illogical thought process that led to the murders of two students fit the profile of prenatal exposure to alcohol, and his mother denies drinking during the pregnancy. Mrs. McLaughlin did not have to contact me, but she did. I admire her courage in doing so.

Red Lake, MN

On a Monday morning, March 21, 2005, in the town of Red Lake on the Red Lake Reservation in northern Minnesota, Jeffery Weise exploded on the world scene with a rampage that had not seen at such a level of carnage by a student since Columbine in 1999. Weise killed his grandfather and his grandfather's significant other. He stole his grandfather's police car, drove it to the school, and then killed a school guard, a teacher and five fellow students. He wounded 15 others. Red Lake Police, who had learned from the hard lesson at Columbine, stormed the school and engaged Weise in gunfire. Knowing his rampage was over, the sixteen-year-old Weise put a shotgun under his chin and pulled the trigger.

The local community was devastated by the attack. Stories of the shooting made headlines nationwide, although access to the community was limited because of the unique sovereign nation status of the Red Lake Nation.

Jeff Weise had a history of behavioral difficulties at the several schools he had attended. He flunked eighth grade and was referred to an alternative school. There, he did not improve academically. He preferred to draw violent pictures and dressed in Goth fashion. He attempted to commit suicide a year before the shootings. He had been expelled from the Red Lake High School months before the shooting and moved to an out of school placement because of his behavioral problems. He was on Prozac for depression and was seeing a therapist. He had alienated his relatives and had a strained relationship with his grandfather.

I immediately realized Jeff Weise suffered from prenatal exposure to alcohol when I saw his facial features on his fourth grade class picture that flashed across the television screen. The physical characteristics of FAS often fade as a person ages and were less evident in his high school pictures. For two years, I had the mistaken understanding the Weise's mother, Joanne, had died shortly after the shooting. When I was informed that wasn't the case, I took on the task of finding Joanne Weise in an effort to confirm what I knew about her son.

It was a clear bright Saturday morning when I drove up to the group home where Joanne Weise lived. She had agreed to talk to me when I called her the previous day. During the call, she confirmed she drank alcohol when she was pregnant with her son Jeff. After I told her of my mission to stop the epidemic of prenatal exposure to alcohol and how her story would be a powerful message to young women, she cautiously said she would be interested in talking with me and agreed to meet.

Joanne Weise's story was revealing. Both of her parents were alcoholic. Joanne grew up in urban Minneapolis area and never lived on the Red Lake reservation. She started drinking when she was sixteen years old, following her parent's footsteps into alcoholism. She became pregnant with Jeff at the age of eighteen and continued drinking throughout the pregnancy. Her son was born about the time the government put warnings labels on alcohol. She had no idea her drinking was damaging her son.

When Jeff was eleven years old, she was severely injured in an alcohol related auto accident. She ended up in long term care for traumatic brain injury. Jeff was sent to live with his grandfather on the Red Lake Reservation after the accident. Never again was she a part of his life.

The first edition of my book had already been out for a couple of months by the time I had this visit. I had read a news article stating she had died as a result of her injuries, and because of that, I had not pursued talking to her. While working with a reporter from the Minneapolis Star Tribune, I found out the information I had was incorrect, which led to me finding her and asking for a visit. Early in the visit I apologized for the mistake, wanting to be completely upfront with her. She graciously accepted my apology.

Joanne's traumatic brain injury was evident. She carefully chose her words and her movements were slow and planned. Her pleasant demeanor and thoughtful conversation made me comfortable in her presence. Here I was, asking her to talk about the most painful time in her life and explaining how her actions when she was pregnant were the root cause for that pain. As she learned more about me, she seemed to become more confident and resolute in her conviction that she needed to help her community by telling her story.

During the visit, she reached into her purse, found what she was looking for and carefully extending her hand, showed me a small silver and blue medallion. She proudly told me she had recently reached her tenth year of sobriety. Then, with humbleness and resolve, she said she needed to tell people her story. Her hand rose to her chest and tapped her heart as she said she wanted to do what she could so another mother did not have to go through the pain she went through. She said she believed this was why God let her live after her accident. I could see the determination in her eyes.

My visit set into motion a plan for her to begin speaking to schools across the state of Minnesota and elsewhere. She was aware, and had now acknowledged, that her actions of so long ago had caused brain damage that became the root cause for her son's actions in Red Lake that fateful morning. By gathering her inner strength and stepping out into the spotlight, she knew she could very well be a catalyst for change in her community and in the world.

Joanne Weise is the first mother of a school shooter to publicly acknowledge that drinking while pregnant had an impact on the actions of her son. Her alcohol related brain injury took her away from her son. Her courage to accept responsibility for her drinking while pregnant is an example for biological mothers worldwide who have prenatally exposed their children to alcohol. Her painfully honest look at her actions is a message to every mother and father as to how devastating prenatal exposure to alcohol can be on the developing fetus.

He clearly exhibited brain damage from prenatal exposure to alcohol by his behaviors in school. His academic and social behaviors, disrupted school experiences, and depression fit the profile of prenatal exposure to alcohol. The fixation on killing as many as he could before he took his own life is an exhibition of the illogical, depressed, brain damaged thinking of a prenatally exposed brain.

Jeff Weise was one of two Native America adolescent males who are categorized as school shooters. In a clear case of bias, the only two mothers of school shooters who were reported as alcoholics by the media were two Native American mothers. If the news reporters were as diligent searching for the truth in the other school shootings, the fatal link would have been established much sooner.

Cazinovia, WI

Less than two years passed before another school shooting occurred in the two states being researched. At 8:00 am, September 29, 2006, Eric Hainstock, a fifteen year-old ninth grade student in Cazenovia, Wisconsin, walked into the high school with his father's handgun and a shotgun. He declared he was going to shoot someone. He aimed the shotgun at a teacher, but a custodian wrestled the gun away from him. Still armed with the handgun, he confronted the principal, John Klang, a well liked and highly respected man in the school and community. Klang had given Hainstock a disciplinary warning a day prior to the shooting for bringing tobacco on school grounds. Klang attempted to disarm Hainstock, and was shot several times. Klang did manage to shove the gun away and wrestle Hainstock to the ground where others helped hold him down. Tragically, John Klang died of his wounds after being airlifted to the University of Wisconsin Hospital in Madison. Hainstock was arrested and charged with intentional homicide, found guilty, and sentenced to life in prison without the possibility of parole for thirty years.

The Cazenovia school shooting provided a wealth of information not found in the earlier shootings. Web forums allowed students who experienced the shooting to share their reactions. This produced a rich source of behavior observations. In addition to the forums, information was gleaned from news reports about the shooting, investigative reports before the trial, and news reports of the trial.

Eric Hainstock suffered through a difficult life. He lived with his dad and stepmother. His father had been charged with abusing him when he was younger. He had been subjected to homophobic remarks at school and according to some was the brunt of teasing and harassment by the "jocks." Website forum participants, identified as friends of Eric, detailed the teasing and harassment Eric endured. Internet forum participants who were classmates of Hainstock, write of bullying and teasing done by Eric, citing instances of him running down the hall pushing everyone out of the way. His classmates tell how he was the perpetrator most of the time. Others tell of how he ate lunch next to Mr. Klang, who had treated him nicely, even to the point of buying Hainstock clothes in times of need.

Eric Hainstock clearly fits the behavior profile of a heavily impacted prenatally exposed child. Students and acquaintances of his family described Eric as a troubled and eccentric child, one who took pride in being in trouble with authority. A friend described him as unstable and dysfunctional. He was diagnosed with a mental disorder and prescribed a psychotropic medication. He was a special education student with an Emotional Behavioral Disability (EBD) label. A student in one of his classes described him as mean. Another described him as a perpetrator. A classmate from elementary school recalled a time when his EBD teacher and an aid carried him from the room while he was tantrumming. Another classmate detailed how he would make sexually inappropriate comments to female teachers. Each of these descriptions of his behaviors by acquaintances and friends confirm the profile of prenatal exposure to alcohol.

This determination is further supported with a comment from an observer who attended Hainstock's murder trial. He stated, "When I saw Eric on the stand, I didn't see evil or malicious. I saw a boy who was very emotionally immature and probably somewhat intellectually immature also." Both observations fit the profile of prenatal exposure.

Eric Hainstock was heavily prenatally exposed to alcohol. His mother had serious problems with alcohol before and during her short marriage to his father. She was pregnant before she got married. After he was born, his parents would take him along to bars while they drank. They divorced in 1993 when Eric was 2 years old. In 1995, a judge stated that both parents had "serious limitations" and he noted the alcohol abuse by the mother. He ordered both parents to stay away from bars and to stop taking Eric to taverns with them. His mother abandoned him and her parental rights were terminated in 2000 after she spent sixty days in jail for non-payment of child support. Soon after, police were informed the then nine year old boy had behavior problems and his father could no longer afford his medication or counseling.

What he did was tragic and undeniably wrong. Most people around him did not know or understand that his brain does not function like yours or mine. He became fixated on the only solution he could control that would resolve the harassment he endured. The harassment included a teacher who made fun of him in front of the gym class for being a special needs student. The discipline for tobacco, rightly and appropriately delivered by Mr. Klang, was another contributing factor. Where a normal brain understands why, his brain works differently or not at all. His brain did not process what would happen when he came to the school threatening to kill someone or what would happen after he pulled the trigger. His brain was incapable of logically linking his actions to a consequence. His brain's executive functions were damaged and he suffered from a lack of judgment as well as limited control of his impulses. When he picked up his father's guns and headed to school, the "Perfect Storm" in his prenatally exposed brain was at full strength. He was the victim of the same fatal link experienced by David Black, Dickie Anderson, Leonard McDowell, Jeff Weise, and Jason McLaughlin.

Jonesboro, AK

Minnesota was the birthplace of another school shooter, Mitchell Johnson. This shooter spent his early formative years living in Grand Meadow, Minnesota. Mitchell Johnson left Minnesota with his mother after she divorced his father. Mitchell Johnson's father still lives in southern Minnesota.

On March 24, 1998, thirteen-year-old Mitchell Johnson and a schoolmate, eleven-year old William Golden, acted on a plan they had concocted to shoot up their school. That morning, Andrew Golden pulled the fire alarm and sent a shiver throughout our nation when he and Mitchell Johnson became the youngest boys ever charged with murder in the nation. They opened fire on the students and teachers as they filed out of the building because of the fire alarm. Five were killed and 10 wounded.

According to news reports, Mitchell Johnson was a contrast in behaviors. One news report said when he was with adults, he acted like a choirboy. The general consensus of reporting showed when he was with kids he was a bully. He was a gang "wannabe", telling kids he was a member of the Bloods, a gang that uses the color red. He had pulled a knife on another student. He threatened students and told them he was going to come to the school and shoot them. Kids reported he was a braggart and a bully. He had a grudge against one of his teachers, Shannon Wright. Reports indicate he told other students he wanted to kill Mrs. Wright.

While Mitchell Johnson was in juvenile detention following the shootings, jailers reported he did not have remorse for his actions and only acted with remorse when his parents were present. Other inmates said he bragged about the shooting, especially the murder of Shannon Wright.

Mitchell Johnson came from a broken home. His dad was much younger than his mother, who was a guard at a federal prison. She was pregnant when they got married. Visitors to their squalid trailer reported there was dog "crap" on the floor, rotting food in the counter, and the yard was not cleaned or mowed. One acquaintance said Mitchell was dirty, his clothes were dirty, and no one wanted their kids to play with him. Locals in Grand Meadow recall his parents running with a rough bunch, riding their motorcycle and being partiers. One local said he "wouldn't want to mess with her" when talking about Mitchell's mother. Another defended her, saying the father was the "runabout" and she was the nice one, but this local did not know anything about her drinking patterns. Mitchell's mother was known to drink alcohol and be a partier when in high school.

While living in Minnesota with his parents, Mitchell would sometimes go for periods of time without parental supervision. Police records indicate law enforcement was called several times to find him. Local law enforcement felt his parents were neglecting him.

His dad was caught stealing from his employer, and soon after, his mother divorced his dad. She later married a tattooed inmate in the prison where she worked as a prison guard. She followed him to Kentucky, then to his hometown of Jonesboro, AK, after his release from prison where he was serving a drug related sentence.

According to a sheriff's report in Minnesota, where he would go to visit his father, Mitchell admitted sexually touching the two-year-old granddaughter of his father's fiancé. Mitchell told authorities that he put his finger inside of her once. Mitch was ordered to undergo psychological counseling.

Johnson's mother fits the profile of drinking during her pregnancy. Mitchell Johnson was born before the government required labels on alcohol containers warning of the dangers of drinking while pregnant. Her low socio-economic status at the time of her pregnancy, being pregnant prior to getting married, her poor parenting, as evidenced by the neglectful supervision and the condition of the house, the fact her spouse was known as a "runabout" and drinker, the reports from the local community regarding her drinking and partying, and as a prison guard, she worked in an environment mostly populated by men, all combine to put her at a very high probability of drinking alcohol when pregnant.

You have most likely heard the details of some of these shootings countless times. What you have not heard in any of the school shootings by any of the experts is the link to the mothers, the link rooted in the brain damage caused by alcohol.

There is a wall of silence around the mothers of school shooters. People close to the family understandably protect the mothers. This normal human response has kept us from the truth. Only in cases of minorities has the major press asked and reported on the behaviors of the mothers. In every case, the focus has been on the student and the student behaviors prior to the shooting, without any focus on the possibility of brain damage from prenatal exposure to alcohol.

CHAPTER Ten

The Dilemma

"**T**his is a Fox News Alert! Nine people are now reported dead in a mass shooting in a shopping mall in Omaha, Nebraska." Another unexplained tragically violent act was being played out on the television screen. The 19-year old-shooter, in what was described as Nebraska's worst mass shooting ever, was portrayed as a troubled youth. His father had, at one time, asked police to arrest him to "scare him straight." He had lost his job at McDonalds for stealing money. He had been treated for ADD and ADHD and depression, and had dropped out of school. His suicide note stated he wanted to go out with style.

I listened and watched to see if anyone asked the question or explored the possibility of prenatal exposure to alcohol. I saw the same television experts espousing behaviors and motives, but not the root cause. I heard one police officer state that it may be impossible to come up with an explanation. Ask me. I will ask the burning question! Please, please, please, ask the question! Was the perpetrator prenatally exposed to alcohol?

Days later, the *Omaha Press*, in a single sentence at the end of an article stated his long gone biological mother was a binge drinker. Once again, no link was drawn between his actions and his mother's drinking.

One evening I watched MSNBC's "The Mind of Manson", a documentary detailing the horrific murders committed by Charles Manson and his band of followers. The program was filled with his lifelong illogical rantings which continued whenever he was in front of a camera or in front of a parole board. As I watched, I wondered if he was another person whose brain was "wired wrong" because of prenatal exposure to alcohol.

An FBI profiler added comment throughout the MSNBC magazine show, bringing the psychological profiling expertise of the highly regarded federal law enforcement agency to the table in the discussion of why Manson did what he did. Her final statement was profoundly wrong. She said the home environment shaped the criminal brain. "Occasionally," she said, "there is a bad seed." She completely missed the most important piece of information.

The answer was hidden, but plain as day, screaming out to the deaf ears of the FBI profiler and MSNBC news reporter. Manson's mother, according to the narrator, was a 17 year-old heavy drinker working the streets. Absolutely no link was made to her drinking while she was pregnant and the resulting brain damage inflicted on her child. Yes, he is a killer, but the simple truth is, he has a brain damage caused by prenatal exposure to alcohol and is not some mystical, romanticized "Hannibal Lector."

The Fatal Link

Four out of six school shooters in Minnesota and Wisconsin, seven murders in an eighteen month span in a small city in Central Minnesota, the Omaha Mall shooting, the list could go on and on. Each of these violent tragic murders was committed by boys and men who were prenatally exposed to alcohol.

This link to the drinking habits of the mother is not unique to Minnesota and Wisconsin. President Bush's Secret Services study of 41 school shooters missed the point. The first shooter named in the Secret Service study, Anthony Barbero, New York, 1974, killed three, wounded eleven, and committed suicide. His mother was alcoholic. This fact was only to be revealed by a relative after she died over 25 years later. In 1997 in Bethel, Alaska, Evan Ramsey killed a student and the principal. His Native American mother was reported to be alcoholic.

In 2007, I began a study of school shooters cumulating in this book. The study evolved from the original hometown shooter to Minnesota shooters, adding Wisconsin shooter, and then the shooters of the Secret Services study. To complete the study, other shooters across the nation were found and analyzed. The sixty-nine total shootings were analyzed in three parts, All Shooters, Secret Services compared to Additional Shooters, and a more intense information gathering on the Minnesota and Wisconsin connected shooters who make up slightly more than 10% of the total number.

Red flags of prenatal exposure to alcohol abound in almost every school shooting case. With the information I could find, of the forty shooters in the Secret Service study (one was unnamed and removed for this study), four shooters did not fit the profile of prenatal exposure to alcohol. Limited or no information could be found in thirteen cases, but twenty-three shooters fit the profile of prenatal exposure to alcohol. **In the Secret Service study cases where I could find enough information detailing the behaviors, school placement, and/or information on the mothers of the shooter, 82% fit the profile of prenatal exposure to alcohol.**

For the Additional Shooters, I looked for cases where the incident happened on school grounds or in a school vehicle. I ruled out any police-reported gang incident or a family violence incident that ended up in school. A total of twenty-three additional shootings and one stabbing (called a shooter for the purposes of simplicity in reporting the study) was analyzed in the study. The five Minnesota and Wisconsin shooters not included in the Secret Services study were added to the Additional Shooters list, for a total of twenty-nine incidents.

The results of the Additional Shooters study mirrored the Secret Services study. Of the twenty-nine shooters, two did not fit the profile. Not enough information could be found on four shooters to make a determination. **In the Additional Shooters cases where enough information could be found, 92% fit the profile of** prenatal exposure to alcohol.

In the more intense study of Minnesota and Wisconsin linked cases, **100% (7) fit the profile, 57% (4) were confirmed to be heavily prenatally exposed to alcohol, 14% (1) had a mother with confirmed binge drinking patterns near to the date of pregnancy, 14% (1) mother denied drinking while pregnant, and 14% (1) did not have enough information on the mother to make a determination.** These are not a fluke statistics. This is the staggering truth: The Fatal Link.

When I started this project, I knew I was going to be making some controversial observations and conclusions. First, I am a white man, learning about this tragic epidemic while working with Native American children and families. I am also a man observing and making statements about something that is inherently a woman's decision.

But, I am a father, a grandfather, and an educator. I am someone who has a stake in this discussion. I am also a taxpayer, someone who is supporting the educational, the social, and the judicial systems, all of which are being overwhelmed by the multitude of victims of the prenatal drinking by expectant mothers. I can't stand by quietly knowing what I know.

This discussion is made even more difficult by the reproductive rights of a woman. Difficult as it may seem, the Supreme Court decision, Roe versus Wade, decided a woman has the right to damage the fetus to the point of death, without repercussion, even if she is carrying the fetus to full-term.

In most states the only protection for the fetus has nothing to do with alcohol, but rather the less damaging drugs, cocaine, crack, or meth. If a mother is using one of those drugs, she can be charged with a felony and put in jail. For the duration of her incarceration, the fetus is not exposed to the drug or to alcohol. Unfortunately, in most states, it is a misdemeanor to provide alcohol to a minor (the fetus in this case), which does not result in a jail sentence. All a woman could be charged with, if caught drunk, is a misdemeanor, which does not result in a jail sentence.

Being incarcerated can have positive consequences. A foster mother sat across the table from me and showed me pictures of four of her foster children from the same family. Three were heavily impacted FASD children, and the fourth, the youngest, was not as impacted. Why? The mother was incarcerated for four months during the pregnancy for a drug related charge. Those four months considerably lessened the prenatal exposure for that child. The investment of the county for the incarceration of the mother will be returned tens of thousand-fold in the money not having to be spent on remediation of the brain damage to the one child that could have happened if she were not in jail. A longitudinal study of that one family should be done over the first 10 years of their lives to show the difference in cost to society for the care of the three heavily brain damaged children versus the lesser brain damaged child, then compared to a child with a healthy brain. A study such as this would show the value of keeping alcoholic women in a non-drinking environment for the length of their pregnancy.

Just as a person does not have the right to exercise free speech by yelling "Fire" in a crowded theater, I strongly believe a woman does not have the right to damage her fetus by drinking alcohol during the pregnancy. I have a hard time justifying the reproductive rights of women in the context of the prenatal exposure to alcohol damage caused to the fetus when exercising that right.

Every right has responsibilities. For the most part, the responsibilities of taking care of the brain damaged children are falling on people other than the ones who exercised their reproductive rights. Currently, no woman that I can find has been held liable for the damage she caused to her child caused by her drinking. Biological mothers deny their culpability. Adoptive parents stagger under the load of raising an FASD child. You only need to read the blogs of adoptive mothers who have taken the responsibility of raising a child damaged by the biological mother's drinking, to understand the extent of the damage. Our entire society is burdened with the responsibilities thrust on it by women exercising their reproductive right to drink when pregnant.

Some states provide some support for pregnant women if they are charged with any alcohol related offense during their pregnancy. Much more needs to be done. The media and government have done a poor job of protecting our society when it comes to prenatal exposure to alcohol. Drugs are a much more sellable story than alcohol.

Our toy industry was almost paralyzed by the revelation of lead in the paint on toys coming from China. Millions, if not billions of dollars were at stake as the toy stores recalled lead painted toys. Factories in China were taken off the list of reputable manufacturers. Broadcasts headlines exploded across our TV screens with the dangers of lead in toys every time a new revelation hit the news.

Lead is a teratogen and the concerns were rightly justified. If only the press would give the same exposure to every new peer-reviewed research study on prenatal exposure to alcohol that every prospective parent needs to hear. Maybe the billions of advertising dollars paid by the alcohol industry limits the media's willingness to tell the story. More disconcerting is the alcohol industries ability to influence our legislators.

I will not give the father of the child a free ride either. Studies are being done to see if there is a genetic link passed on by alcohol damaged sperm. My research indicates a grave responsibility on the part of the male partner in the relationship to help the mother refrain from drinking. Far too many times the man encourages the expectant mother to drink and is therefore equally culpable.

Our culture does not recognize the importance of refraining from drinking during a pregnancy. Coors Beer has a commercial that starts like any ordinary beer commercial. The guy walks to the fridge, picks up a beer and gets excited when the mountain on the bottle label turns blue. The female partner then bursts out of the bathroom, excitedly showing him the pregnancy test that has turned blue. He doesn't care about her pregnancy, only the cold beer. This reveals a basic societal problem. Of course, the point of the commercial is to advertise beer. I found making fun of a pregnancy with a beer commercial to be repugnant. My tirade on YouTube went as such:

What gives, Coors Brewing Company? Do any of you know that drinking any alcohol any time during of the pregnancy, after the zygote becomes a fetus, will damage the brain of the fetus? How can you, as a reputable corporation, make a commercial that celebrates a cold beer while making fun of a pregnancy? Anyone who has any understanding of the damage drinking during a pregnancy can cause would know the man in the commercial should have immediately taken all the beer out of the house so the mother did not have anyone influencing her to drink any alcohol. Another inference I make is the mother probably drank your beer prior to knowing she was pregnant, and, in that case, has already damaged the brain of the unborn child. Instead, your commercial makes fun of the mother. Your message minimizes a pregnancy in a situation I would suggest is ripe for the man influencing the mother to drink. Anytime his addiction to your product is more important than the life he brings into the world, the loser is the child.

The comments on this display of emotion ranged from very supportive to:

Really this is the only thing you can complain about?

And the video did change minds. Here is the script of a series of posts from one viewer.

I think maybe you missed the point; it was a joke. It was also quite funny. I agree that a woman shouldn't be drinking while pregnant but, I don't think your paranoia is going to curb it, certainly not through YouTube. I think that could have just as easily been a coke commercial, or a sports commercial with another twist. Calm down. Drink a beer. Write a letter to someone who might actually listen to you seriously. Then, drink another beer. You'll probably feel better.

After a few exchanges, the person who made the above comment revealed he was personally affected by prenatal exposure to alcohol, but did not realize he was until he made that flippant comment about the Coors Beer video.

I'm a cop, and I see what people do to their children all the time. I had a little bro born preemie b/c my mom drank while pregnant.

Don't take my sarcasm or less-than-polite jest as good reason to be bitter. There are much more tragic things in the world going on to protest and fight against, like abortion, starving children in our own country, lax laws on child predators, child abuse, stem-cell research, etc... Let a dumb (though funny) joke be just that. Don't be uncomfortable w/ laughing.

A couple more exchanges and he had a totally different tenor to his post.

I would like to pick your brain more about the subject, have very briefly read up on it on your site and a couple of others now, but am not entirely satisfied, and may or may not have an argument of my own (I say my own - probably not) or points to test. Thanks for the info and insight.

I observed a couple in a local Wisconsin bar where I had gone to gather information on the Tomah shooting. She came into the bar drinking a Mountain Dew, obviously pregnant. He was so drunk he was having a hard time talking. Situations such as this take an enormous amount of willpower on the part of the expectant mother to refrain from just one drink, which leads to two, three, and more and the circle continues. The father of the child has the responsibility to not put the expectant mother in that situation for the term of the pregnancy, and, if they are planning a pregnancy, to make sure she does not drink during the time they are trying to become pregnant.

I do not write this book to shame mothers who exposed their children to alcohol. My motive is to stop this epidemic. If I have made someone angry with my observations, I accept that. If this takes exposing the drinking patterns of mothers to reach this goal, so be it. If every child can only enroll in school after the mother provides a response to a question about drinking during the pregnancy, I support that.

If every time a police officer arrests a suspect, he or she is questioned about his or her mother's drinking habits, we might get closer to the truth. If we incentivize pregnancies to ensure an alcohol free pregnancy, the cost of the incentives for a healthy brain would have a payback of millions of dollars.

This is too important a subject to keep hidden under the cloak of guilt. I will not change my message to pacify someone who is worried about the "cultural trauma" of the Native American people, or the guilt of the mothers. I cry inside every time I see another child, no matter what ethnic or socioeconomic background, so damaged he or she will never have a normal life, all because of the selfish desires of or ingnorance of the mother and, in my opinion, in many cases, the even more selfish alcoholic and sexual motives of the father.

The warnings are there. Every alcohol container warns of the dangers. Every woman who drinks while pregnant is walking a tightrope of chance. She may think she can make it through with no damage to the child, but one binge, one time where a couple beers are drunk quickly without food in her stomach, one or two glasses of wine a day to calm the nerves, a family occasion, a wedding party, a night out with the girls, and she falls off that tightrope without knowing the damage that is happening to the little life inside.

Her baby looks so perfect, has all the fingers and toes, a full head of hair, and so seemingly fine. Not until first grade, when the child struggles with linking a sound to a symbol, or has trouble sounding out a three letter word while the rest of the class is moving on to consonant blends, will the truth be known. She won't know until the temper tantrums escalate, or the impulsive behaviors impede learning, or the her child's inability to attend to a task brings calls from the teacher. That perfect looking child will then reveal the brain damage from that one binge, that party, that forgotten weekend, or that two glasses of wine a day, as the ABC television report glorified. And, if our awareness of this silent epidemic does not change, the culprit will remain hidden behind the cloak of ignorance.

When I have tried to control my eating habits, I have lied to myself many times about the number of times a day I have sneaked a piece of candy or snatched one of the chocolate bars a teacher or student brought in to my office as a treat. Only when I would take the time to chart what I ate did I really take inventory of my dietary cheating. Unfortunately, the same forgetfulness and denial happens to people who have been in the habit of drinking throughout their lives.

Denial is habitual for people with a drinking habit. Forgetting the amount a person drank over the course of nine months is common. Forgetting how many drinks a person had in one setting is common. Lying to the doctor about drinking is more common than you would think.

There are as many perceptions and definitions of "drinking" as there are numbers of diets. I quickly learned to define the question in more clinical terms. I now ask the question in a couple of ways: "Did the mother drink <u>any</u> alcohol while pregnant?" or, "Did the mother expose the fetus to <u>any</u> alcohol?" I only ask the question when the persistent behavioral clues are evident. A 'yes' answer to the question immediately places the child into the category of potential brain damage. Any time the answer is no, but the child displays classic behaviors of brain damage, I will chose to let the behaviors be a stronger indication than the denial, until I am convinced otherwise.

The time between conception and the realization of being pregnant exposes 25% to 30% of fetuses to alcohol. Women, who would never drink if they knew they were pregnant, unwittingly can do damage the fetus to the point of the full syndrome because they don't know they are pregnant.

A professional woman engaged me in a conversation in the church basement. She knew I spoke on FASD. Here was someone you would never think would drink while pregnant, a well respected professional in every way, knowledgeable about the dangers of drinking while pregnant, and working with children who exhibited behaviors reflective of prenatal exposure.

She confided to me her story of an unplanned pregnancy and the social drinking she was doing with her husband and friends prior to finding out about her pregnancy. She spoke of her shock upon finding out she was pregnant and her concerns for her child. This is a common story, unplanned pregnancy and drinking during child-bearing years. We need more than education, but will more education stop this dilemma?

The mothers of the school shooters across the nation did not know their drinking would result in brain damage. They did not know they contributed to their sons taking guns to school and becoming murderers. If they did, they would probably not have drunk a single drop. This is not about mothers wanting to harm their child. This is about warning mothers regarding the consequences of drinking while pregnant, in an attempt to stop the carnage.

Even if every mother stopped drinking during her pregnacy today, we would still have another generation of brain damaged children moving through our educational system. The school systems would not see the results healthy brains for five years or more. It would take fifteen years to see a drop in school shootings. Healthy brains do not commit school shootings.

The professionals working with children exhibiting the behaviors of brain damage need to learn and understand the root cause. Professionals need to move past the fear of embarrassing or shaming the mother. They need to move past unsubstantiated denials of drinking in order to make an accurate diagnosis of the behaviors exhibited by the child and, in my opinion, to realize how much this is impacting our society. I have long since stopped worrying if I am making the parents feel guilty by asking the question. I have actually found the opposite to be true. Mothers and fathers have been relieved to find out the root cause and have requested more information.

Psychologists and doctors make a mistake that contributes to the dilemma. Many make the assumption the behaviors of the child are genetically passed from the parents. Parents explain they had the same characteristics when they were a child. In my experience, the parents were explaining their own FASD behaviors. No one thought to ask them if the parents mother's drank. The behaviors thought to be genetic are, in many or most cases, evidence of the generation after generation of brain damage caused by prenatal exposure to alcohol.

For many years working on reservations, I thought I was working where the abnormal had become normal, where children with brain damage were the norm, rather than children with healthy brains. I now see we are all living where the abnormal has become normal. Our entire society has been impacted with this epidemic to the extent we think it is normal that a quarter of our children will have problems reading and math. We think it is normal we have violence and crime. We think it is normal one out of five children have mental illness, depression, and are medicated with Ritalin and other psychotropic drugs. This is not normal. We live where the abnormal has become normal!

The greatest dilemma is the fact that much of the brain damage occurs without any physical deformities. The child looks perfect, all fingers and toes are there, perfect symmetry to the face and body, and no indication of the atrophy of the brain. This hidden damage is fooling professionals and parents. A shield of ignorance, almost impenetrable, due to the unwillingness to confront the truth, protects the alcohol industry. We are condemning another generation of unborn with the message that only massive drinking causes harm. If you don't see the damage, no harm done. Wrong.

CHAPTER Eleven
The Solution

E ric's father was a military man. He was an Air Force pilot, a job
that is notorious for hard partying. At his 20th class reunion, he
answered the question "What I like?" with: "Eating, drinking, flying
and loving, not necessarily in that order." They were a typical Air
Force family serving our nation with pride and commitment.

Eric's parents had a church wedding at a First Presbyterian Church
on April 17, 1970. Eric was born well before the public awareness of
the dangers of drinking during pregnancies, a full seven years before
warnings were placed on all alcohol. His mother, like so many mothers
of that generation, would have never taken a drink of alcohol when
pregnant if she knew the dangers. She stayed home when Eric was
young; keeping busy with military wives luncheons, volunteer projects
and school functions, providing by all accounts, a fine strong normal
upbringing for her family. Their children grew up in this highly
structured, caring, nurturing home, playing sports and doing family
outings, a typical Air Force family in their neighborhood.

Despite the good environment of the home and the excellent
upbringing by the parents, the clues are there. The family was

Presbyterian, a denomination that does not demand abstinence from alcohol. He was born before mothers were warned about the dangers of drinking while pregnant. His parents were in a high risk, high stress occupation, with an active social life. They had to move when the job demanded it. His dad's answer to his class reunion question indicates alcohol was a part of their lives. Behaviors, not publicly displayed while Eric was young, started to become visible as he moved into adolescence when the high family structure of his younger years lessened.

Eric Harris' behaviors were deviant enough to come to the attention of the sheriff's office. According to court papers, the sheriff's office had been told that he had threatened to kill another student. After being arrested for theft, Harris was remanded to a juvenile diversion project in Jefferson County. In documents filled out in his diversion program, Harris' own words in some of the diversion documents state, for example: "Short temper, often get angry at almost anything I don't like, like people I have no respect for trying to tell me what to do. People telling me what to think. I have too many inside jokes or thoughts to have very many friends. I hate too many things."

He noted that he experienced anger, anxiety, depression, disorganized thoughts, homicidal thoughts, jealousy, loneliness, mood swings, obsessive thoughts, racing thoughts, stress, suspiciousness, and a temper.

His illogical thinking and displays of anger and depression, which culminated in a psychiatric diagnosis needing the medication Luvox, are clues. The brush with the law resulting in a charge of theft and a sentence to an anger management class is a clue. But his clothing hid the most significant clue, something to which no attention was given by the profilers and pundits; a peculiar physical characteristic that was viewed as an abnormal trait without significance.

This clue is a physical characteristic of a birth defect caused by prenatal exposure to alcohol, a concave chest. Eric did not want to remove his T-shirt in gym class because this physical feature caused teasing from his peers. This feature would haunt him throughout his short life and is the one clue that solidifies the probability of his being prenatally exposed to alcohol.

Eric Harris was planning to follow his dad's example of service to the country by becoming a United States Marine. When he did not tell the truth about his medication on his application, the Marine Corps rejected it, setting into motion his plans for the worst high school massacre in the United States, Columbine, Littleton, CO.

How many adolescents who fit this profile go to your child's school? Is there a way of finding out?

Canada is far ahead of the United States when it comes to recognizing the epidemic of Fetal Alcohol Spectrum Disorders. The Diagnostic and Statistical Manual of Mental Disorders (DSM), the bible for American psychologists, does not recognize FASD as a mental illness in the United States, while the Canadian manual does. Most of the FASD behaviors are classified in one way or another, such as Reactive Attachment Disorder, or Attention Deficit Hyperactivity Disorder, and Autism. Without a classification, FASD remains a shadow, an unrecognizable, mostly denied, root cause, shoved into the background and not asked about or discussed by the great majority of mental health professionals.

Prenatal exposure to alcohol is, by far, the single greatest cause of mental retardation, stunted social skills, and arrested emotional development. Prenatal exposure to alcohol is America's greatest brain drain.

I can see only one solution to completely eradicate this entirely preventable epidemic. This solution will take the partnership of the beverage industry and the government.

I challenge the alcohol industry to develop a tasteless additive to their products that interacts with the chemical changes in a woman's body when she becomes pregnant, causing the woman to regurgitate the alcohol.

This is doable if the political will is there. Education will not change an alcoholic's behavior. Posters will not change the binge drinking of young women. Awareness will not change the drinking habits of unknowlingly pregnant women. If we really want to have healthy brains for children, we need to protect the fetus from any and all alcohol.

Until this happens, we will always be reactive. Children will continue to be exposed to alcohol in utero. Mothers will expose children before they know they are pregnant. Alcoholic mothers and alcohol-drinking mothers will continue to drink, bringing an exponentially greater number of children into our world with brain damage.

This solution is pro-active. For the little percentage of time a woman can't drink, the pay-off for our society will be tremendous.

If this is not a solution embraced by the alcohol industry, I propose the victims of the next school shooting investigate the drinking habits of the mother of the shooter and file civil suits against the makers of her favorite beers, hard liquors and wines. The alcohol industry has made no attempt to limit pregnant women from damaging their children. They could do so much more.

Most likely, the industry will need to be hit in the pocketbook for them to do more than put a hard-to-read warning label in the most inconspicuous location on the beverage container. I hope not, but I believe change will only happen when the alcohol industry, like the tobacco industry, has to pay out billions of dollars to pay for the damage caused by their products.

Until such time as science can find a solution,

I challenge the alcohol industry to actively inform the public about the dangers of drinking while pregnant and to support programs with that message.

What can we do?

- **Remember, every drink when pregnant has the potential to take potential from the developing fetus.**
- Educate ourselves.
- Both the mother and father bear responsibility for the health of the fetus.
- Fathers need to know the dangers of FASD and refrain from putting the expectant mother into situations where drinking may happen.
- Women in their childbearing years need to know that brain damage to the developing fetus will result from alcohol consumption and to not drink any alcohol when any possibility of a pregnancy could occur.

- Doctors need to continually tell every expectant mother to completely refrain from alcohol.
- Doctors need to have the training and courage to identify prenatally exposed children as early as possible.
- Every pregnant mother should be tested for alcohol use regularly throughout the pregnancy.
- Insurance providers must require doctors to test urine and hair samples of every pregnant woman and the meconium of the newborns for prenatal exposure to alcohol. The results must be entered into the permanent medical records of the child.
- Teachers need to understand the brain damage caused by FASD and the need to impress on students the dangers of drinking during pregnancy before the students reach childbearing age.
- Shaming and blaming and other similar behaviors by educational personnel and adults need to stop.
- Parents need to be diligent in setting an example, as well as being specific with their children about the dangers of drinking during a pregnancy.
- Parents must insist their school administrators learn about the profile of school shooters and look within their student population for students who fit the profile.
- The clergy must lead in delivering the message without religious overtones.
- Laws must be changed to protect the fetus without interfering with the reproductive rights of the mother.
- Litigation against alcohol producing companies needs to be initiated to bring this issue to the forefront.
- The insurance industry needs to provide incentives, using frequent testing, to ensure alcohol free pregnancies.
- Law enforcement personnel need to ask the question of prenatal exposure with every arrest and keep the statistics.
- As a society, we need to have the expectation that drinking during a pregnancy is absolutely, without exception, unacceptable.
- And, in order to uncover the magnitude of this epidemic, whenever juvenile and adult deviant and/or violent behavior happens, we must always ask the question, "Did the mother drink ANY alcohol during the pregnancy?"

The alcohol industry and government need to take responsibility for this growing epidemic. The limited educational initiatives, undertaken by well-meaning, but underfunded non-profits organizations devoted to informing the public, only serve as a finger in the hole in the dam. We need to stop the flood of damaged children overwhelming our special educations programs, our schools, our social services, our jails, our communities, and our nation. We need to break the Fatal Link.

Addendum One of Two

I am adding this addendum and asking for help. I have conducted a FASD probability study, looking at the behaviors of the shooter and family, looking for clues that place the shooter on or remove the shooter from the probability of prenatal exposure to alcohol. You can help by providing me with information. If one of these shootings happened in your town or city, in your school, or was committed by someone in your family, and you have information on the mother of the shooter, you can contact me at jodycrowe@gmail.com. I will be continuing this study to further confirm whether the mother prenatally exposed these shooters.

If any violent, deviant act happens in your community and you know the perpetrator was prenatally exposed to alcohol, let me know. We need to expose these completely preventable tragedies and stop this from happening in the future.

Study of School Shooters for the
Probability of Prenatal Exposure to Alcohol

Abstract

This research is a study of the probability of brain damage from prenatal exposure to alcohol in the fatal school shootings in the United States, from 1966 to September 2008. A total of sixty-eight shooters and one stabbing were studied. There were 67 males and 2 females in the study. The study is in two parts, the macro being a study of all 69 of the perpetrator's behaviors and their mother's drinking behaviors. A study within the study is of the six school shooters in Minnesota and Wisconsin, along with one school shooter who was born in Minnesota. Forty of the forty-one school shooters in the Secret Services study are included. One Secret Service study shooter was not named and was removed from the list for this study.

This study is not being funded by any organization or outside person. The author has conducted this study for the purposes of alerting the public as to the depth of the problem caused by prenatal exposure to alcohol and to educate educators and other professionals as to why every student, both male and female, should fully understand the dangers of drinking alcohol when pregnant.

Method

Behaviors of both the perpetrator and perpetrator's family were found by researching newspapers, web posts, and blogs. Letters were sent to principals, shooters, people identified in newspaper articles as knowing the shooter, victims' families, parents and relatives of the shooters, and law enforcement officers identified in some cases. People were interviewed who had personal knowledge of the perpetrator's history, including family members when possible. Emails were sent when addresses could be found. Inquiries were sent to contact people on some shooter support web pages. Historical societies and public libraries in some towns were visited and historical records were copied. In other cases, historical societies were contacted for information.

The data was gathered. Web pages, news reports, blogs and web posts were stored digitally. Notes were taken and logged for interviews and phone conversations. All correspondence was filed for future reference.

The Five Factors Used to Determine Probability

Five factors were considered when determining the probability of prenatal exposure. The data for each shooter was analyzed to find words, key phrases, school placement, and actions that described or portrayed the shooter and shooter's family. The amount of data for each shooter varied greatly. In some cases, determination was made using a few words that implied behaviors. In other cases, there were news story upon news story detailing behaviors. The five factors used are as follows:

Mother and Family of Subject

The first factor is the factual information on the mother and family. Research into the drinking habits of women of childbearing years provided determiners such as age, social status, smoking habits, work history and drinking habits of spouse. Three determiners are added as a result of my observations. They are church affiliation, a traumatic event during the pregnancy and whether the perpetrator lived with his biological mother and was not adopted. A denial of drinking during a pregnancy is given less weight than observed drinking behaviors by the mother or a pattern of drinking in the family.

A clear unequivocal statement of absolutely no alcohol consumption during the pregnancy immediately removes FASD as a possible diagnosis. (found in only one case) The behaviors would then be a result of biological or environmental factors in the perpetrator's life other than prenatal exposure to alcohol. If there is no information regarding the mother, the probability of FASD remains. Assumptions are made with a researched probability applied to the information given.

Behaviors of Subject

The second determiner is the academic and social behaviors of the individual. The behaviors displayed by the damaged brain can vary to such a degree a combination of as few as three behaviors could indicate a high probability of FASD. Behaviors used to determine probability are directly linked by research to fetal exposure to alcohol. Some behaviors receive more weight as the research indicates higher percentages of FASD victims exhibit these behaviors. This determiner has more factors than the other three due to the spectrum of behaviors exhibited by FASD victims.

A news report stating a shooter was on the "Honor Roll" did not preclude the shooter being determined as High Probability. Honor Roll and Honor Student are hard to quantify without specific classes and grades. A special education student would be getting A's and B's, but not be working at grade level.

Words such as troubled, difficult student, etc, were used quite often in news reports. These words are the red flags of academic and social behavior problems and were used to determine placement on the probability tool.

The act of bringing a gun to school and committing a murder adds weight to the probability scale in the area of judgment and executive function of the brain in all cases. In some cases, the actions of the shooter before, during, and after the shooting are identified and calculated in the determination of probability of prenatal exposure to alcohol.

Behavior Based Diagnosis

Diagnoses by psychologists or psychiatrist make up the third determiner. ADHD/ADD, Autism, Reactive Attachment Disorder (RAD), Obsessive Compulsive Disorder (OCD), Pervasive Development Disorder (PDD), Asperger Syndrome, Tourettes Syndrome, Oppositional Defiant Disorder, and Conduct Disorders have been linked by research to prenatal exposure to alcohol. A prescribed psychotropic medication implied a diagnosis brought on by behaviors that would determine High Probability.

Secondary Disabilities

The fourth determiner is the development of secondary disabilities, such as depression, mental illness, trouble with the law, exposure to violence, and disrupted school experience, that are brought on by the surrounding environmental factors. Societal responses to behaviors, such as special education services, alternative school placements, and trouble with the law resulting in incarceration are factors. Research by Dr. Anne Streissguth and my personal observations, are the basis for this factor.

As an educator, I have a great deal of experience with behaviors that result in the removal of students from the mainstream schools and into alternative schools. Federal law mandates students are to be placed in the least restrictive environment, which means students, by law, have the right to be in the mainstream classroom. The student either chose to be placed in an alternative setting, their parents demanded an alternative setting, or they displayed behaviors that required a more restrictive placement. Most students are placed or encouraged to move to the alternative setting rather than choose to be placed in that setting.

Most students who are removed to alternative schools fit the academic and behavioral profile of prenatal exposure to alcohol because they display the secondary disabilities of FASD. Truancy, suspensions, expulsions, dropping out of school, violence, threatening behaviors, drug and alcohol use, and highly disruptive behaviors are common reasons for alternative school placements. School report cards showing academic achievement reveal great discrepancies between mainstream schools and alternative schools for behaviorally challenged students. The academic records of alternative schools fit the profile of schools with FASD students. Most alternative schools have very high rates of special education students. Some only have high service EBD students. In the study of school shooters, any student who had been or was enrolled in an alternative setting was determined to fit the profile.

The school shooting was a criminal act, which is a component of the secondary disabilities factor. The crime also causes a disruption of school, another component of the secondary disabilities factor. Neither, in itself or combined, causes a determination of probability of prenatal exposure, but the act adds weight to the determination.

Physical Characteristics

The fifth determiner scores any physical characteristics of FASD. This factor is more definitive, but not required for a probable determination. Only a small percentage of FASD victims show physical evidence and aging diminishes the distinctive physical characteristics of many FASD victims.

The Analysis of the Shooters

A Canisius College, Buffalo, NY team of professors and research assistants examined archival resources from school, court and mental health records; accounts from the attackers' personal journals; interviews with school personnel; and FBI records. They found a cluster of four behavior patterns of the typical school shooter. The typical shooter had very low self-esteem, suffered feelings of alienation, lacked resiliency and was bullied. The study found that 67% of school shooters had turbulent relationships with their parents. More than 70% lacked parental support, supervision or discipline. Furthermore, 87% of the shooters lacked resiliency, 73% felt alienated, 67% demonstrated poor coping skills, and 53% showed signs of depression. A total of 67% were bullied, 60% were involved in a deviant peer group, and 33% used drugs or alcohol. Furthermore, 67% experienced turbulent parental relationships. Did they look for prenatal exposure to alcohol? No.

Forensic specialists suggest that the school killer is an avenger, with a rigid cognitive style characterized by all-or-nothing thinking, bored by normal adolescent past times, likely to come from homes where the prevailing emotion is anger and hostility and the mode of discipline is harsh and inconsistent. They often have a personal history of temper tantrums and deep sibling rivalries, a "my life sucks attitude" that is also suspicious of others' motives, lacking a stable self image, and likely to engage in more deviant sexual practices. (McGee, J.P. and DeBernardo, C.R., 1999). Once again, the study is looking at the behaviors from a reactive position and not looking for a root cause.

Eldin Taylor (1999) writes, "Historically the school shooter is a loner who comes from a smaller community. He has been ridiculed by classmates, peers and family. He senses a lack of love and an intolerability of existence. He may suffer an affective disorder and find himself unable to bond with others. His moods may vacillate between bi-polar absolute worthlessness and a super superior form of self-aggrandizement." I couldn't have said it better, unless I added, "brought on by the brain damage of prenatal exposure to alcohol."

Following the Columbine tragedy, President Bush ordered a Secret Services report on school shooters, as I stated previously in the book. The resulting report identified many factors that contributed to the spate of school shooters, but did not indicate a link between shooters other than all were boys. The reason all were boys is because they only selected boys to study. Unfortunately, this report did not ask the right questions.

The following are lists of the shooters researched by the Secret Services and other shooters in an Additional Shooters list. Only 40 of the 41 shooters on the Secret Service list could be researched because one was unnamed. Since the Secret Service study included on Wisconsin shooter, the five Minnesota and Wisconsin shooters are added into the Additional Shooter list for a total of sixty-eight shooters and one perpetrator who used a knife. The resulting probability for prenatal exposure to alcohol is provided for each shooter where there was enough information to do an analysis.

Only with the two Native American shooters did reporters publicly report the mother's drinking patterns. Only in a few other cases were references to mothers' drinking were found after significant research. As expected, the majority of mothers were portrayed as grieving mothers and little or no attempt was made to do any investigative reporting on the mother.

This study disaggregated the shooters into pre-1994, post 1994. The news reporting on line was significantly better post 1994. Years ago, young shooters were given juvenile protection under the law, so information was harder to find. This disaggregating was done to determine if there was a difference in relevant information and if that difference impacted the validity of the data from earlier shootings.

The study also disaggregated the shooters by age using sixteen years of age as the divider. The hypothesis was younger students were more likely to fit the profile of prenatal exposure to alcohol.

Forty of the forty-one shooters studied by the Secret Service were disaggregated from twenty-eight other shooters and one stabbing.

Results of the Study

The study was done in three stages. The Secret Services list of shooters was researched and analyzed as a separate list. The second list was identified as Additional Shooters. Finally, the Minnesota and Wisconsin were analyzed in a more detailed manner and added to the Additional Shooters list for the purposes of the comprehensive study.

Total number of:

- violent incidents in study - 69
- shooters in combined study - 68
- stabbings in the combined study – 1
- males in combined study – 67
- females in combined study – 2

Enough information was found in 66% of the total combined cases to make a determination of probability of pre-natal exposure to alcohol. Not enough information could be found for 25% of the shooters in the combined list. A determination was made that the shooter did not fit the profile of prenatal exposure to alcohol in 9% of the cases. (see Figure 1)

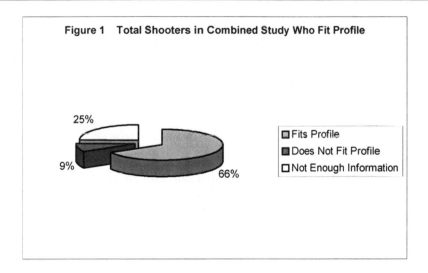

Figure 1 Total Shooters in Combined Study Who Fit Profile

25%

9%

66%

☐ Fits Profile
■ Does Not Fit Profile
☐ Not Enough Information

In the combined study, 88% of the school shooters fit the profile of prenatal exposure to alcohol when enough information was found to make a determination. (see Figure 2)

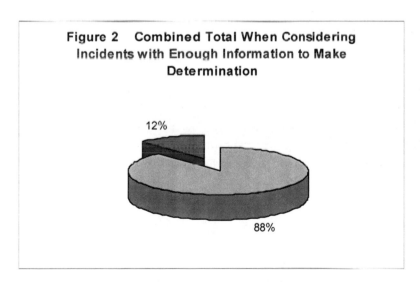

Figure 2 Combined Total When Considering Incidents with Enough Information to Make Determination

12%

88%

In Figure 3, the study shows a smaller percentage of shooters prior to 1994 fit the profile when enough information was found. Information on Pre-1994 shooters was difficult to find and was usually taken from compiled lists using common information. The possibility of prenatal exposure to alcohol for every shooter Pre-94 is over 50% because every shooter was born prior to the government warnings place on alcoholic beverages and before much information on the danger of drinking while pregnant was disseminated through the media. The percentage in Figure 3 could easily be higher if more information were readily available.

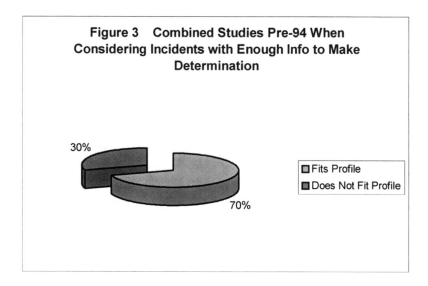

Figure 3   Combined Studies Pre-94 When Considering Incidents with Enough Info to Make Determination

Figure 4 shows the information gap that is a reality of the shooting events prior to 1994. This is because the internet was not a media source prior to the 1990's and the laws were stricter on dissemination of information about juveniles.

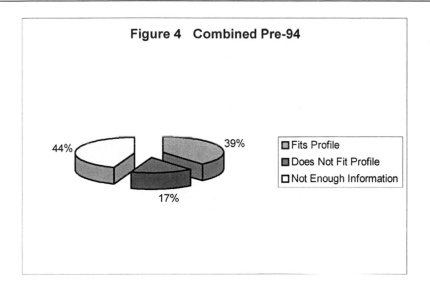

Figure 4   Combined Pre-94

More information could be found for the shooters who were not on the Secret Service list. There were more non-fatal shootings on the Secret Service list. Very little information could be found for the non-fatal incidents in the Secret Service study. (see Figure 5)

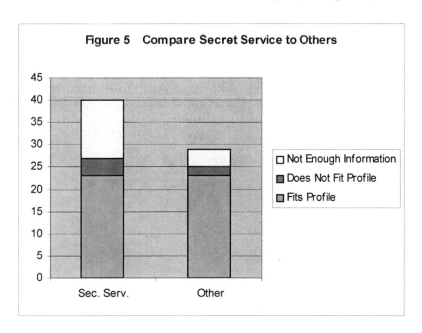

Figure 5   Compare Secret Service to Others

When looking at the over/under 16 data, less information was available on the younger shooters, most likely because of restrictions on information because of juvenile laws. (see Figure 6)

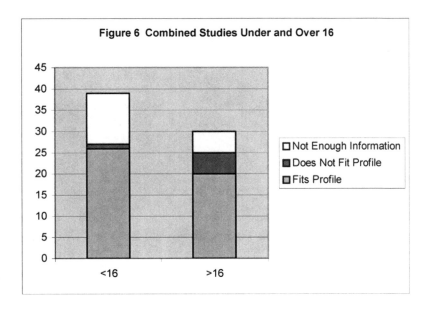

In the combined study, (Figure 7) eight shootings prior to 1994 were non-fatal. Of the eight non-fatal incidents, not enough information to make a determination of probability occurred in five cases. News reports were found, but very little background information was reported on the shooter or shooter's family. In 50% of the under 16 cases, enough information could be found, which suggests a higher curiosity by news reporters when the younger shooter committed the crime, even though juvenile records were protected by law. This was before under-age school shooters were being prosecuted as adults.

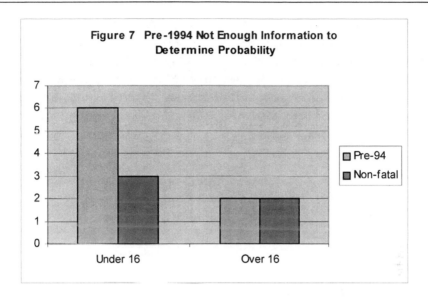

In the combined study (Figure 8), the rate of shooters in which not enough information could be gathered remained about the same after 1994. Information was scarce when a shooting did not result in a fatality.

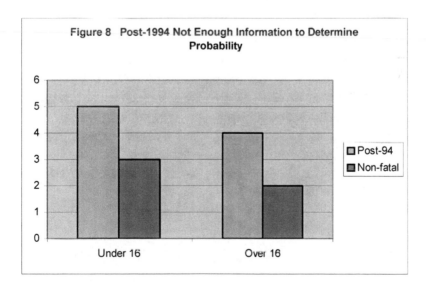

The internet played a part in greater access to information on the shooter, as evidenced in Figure 9. Data sources included media websites, blogs, forums, and archives of historical information. The combined total percentage of Post-94 shooters who fit the profile is 93% compared to 70% of the Pre-94 shooters. This significant difference could be due to the difference in information sharing between the two time spans. If the same type of information were available for the Pre-94 shooters, the percentage fitting the profile would most likely increase.

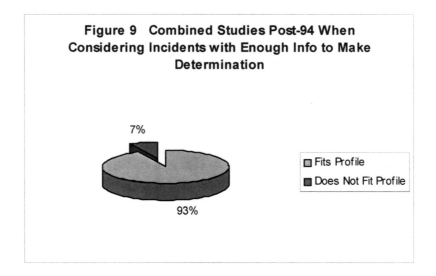

Figure 9   Combined Studies Post-94 When Considering Incidents with Enough Info to Make Determination

In Figure 10, all seven of the shooters from Minnesota and Wisconsin fit the profile of prenatal exposure to alcohol. No information could be found on the mother of the 21 year old Wisconsin adult with significant mental illness issues. The mothers of two shooters were confirmed to be binge drinkers near to the time of their pregnancies. Four shooters were confirmed to have heavy prenatal exposure to alcohol.

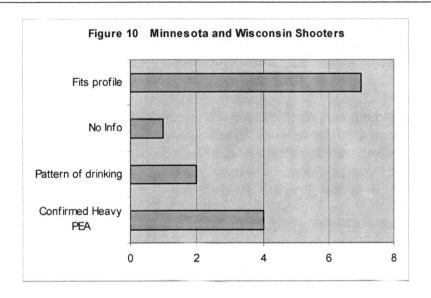

Figure 10   Minnesota and Wisconsin Shooters

The Secret Service Study of School Shooters List

1. Anthony Barbaro, 18, Olean, N.Y., Dec. 30, 1974.

Anthony Barbaro brought guns and homemade bombs to Olean High School, set off the fire alarm, and shot at janitors and firemen who responded. After less than two hours, he had killed three and wounded eleven. A SWAT unit captured him. He hanged himself while awaiting trial.

According to what was reported, Tony was an intelligent boy. Some of his friends reported he had been writing about blowing up the school since he was 10 years old. These same friends had never been invited to his house because Tony said his parents did not like strangers in the house. One friend wrote he thought things were "not cool" in the house. His family was Catholic, a church that does not view drinking alcohol as a moral issue. His mother was an alcoholic, reported by Tony's cousin following the death of Tony's mother. He fits the profile of FASD when the IQ score is high, but the FASD brain damage effects judgment and emotions.

Fits Profile   Pre-1994   Fatal   >16

2. John Christian, 13, Austin, Texas, May 19, 1978.

John Christian, an honor student, shot and killed one of his teachers. There is very little information on this shooting. He was the son of George Christian, former press secretary to President Johnson.

Christian was born before there was any knowledge of the damage caused by alcohol. There is over a 50% chance he was prenatally exposed to alcohol using the statistics of drinking habits of women in their childbearing years.

Not Enough Info Pre-1994 Fatal   <16

3. Robin Robinson, 13, Lanett, Ala., Oct. 15, 1978.

There is little information to be easily obtained on this shooting due to the fact the shooting did not end in a fatality.

Robinson was born before there was any knowledge of the damage caused by alcohol. There is over a 50% chance he was prenatally exposed to alcohol using the statistics of drinking habits of women in their childbearing years.

Not Enough Info   Pre-1994   Non-Fatal   < 16

4. James Alan Kearbey, 14, Goddard, Kan., Jan. 21, 1985.

Kearbey walked into the Junior High School in Goddard Kansas and opened fire, killing the popular Junior High School Principal and wounded two teachers and one student. New York Times reported him as a troubled youth. Reports said he was bullied and beaten by students for years. James Alan Kearbey, 14 years old, was charged with first-degree murder. A teacher said the youth was a loner with a quick temper who was fascinated by weapons. Classmates often teased the teen-ager, several people said, and recently had been beaten by two students in a locker-room fight, according to a neighbor.

Kearbey was born before there was any knowledge of the damage caused by alcohol. The reports stating he was a troubled youth and had a quick temper further raise the probability he was FASD. There is over a 50% chance he was prenatally exposed to alcohol using the statistics of drinking habits of women in their childbearing years.

Fits Profile   Pre-1994   Fatal   < 16

5. Kristofer Hans, 14, Lewiston, Mont., Dec. 4, 1986.

Hans was known to be a bright student, but he had changed when he moved to his freshman year. He was known to be shy. He started losing friends. He was failing French, and had threatened to kill the French teacher, but the French teacher was not in school the day he brought the gun. He killed the substitute teacher instead. Injured a vice principal and two students.

Hans was born before there was any knowledge of the damage caused by alcohol. There is over a 50% chance he was prenatally exposed to alcohol using the statistics of drinking habits of women in their childbearing years.

Not Enough Info   Pre-1994   Fatal   < 16

6. Nathan Faris, 12, DeKalb, Mo., March 2, 1987.

Faris was reportedly teased about his chubbiness. He shot a classmate three times, killing him, after the schoolmate tried to wrestle the gun away from him. He then shot himself to death.

He had a very strict religious home life. A friend reported that he was not happy with his home life. This was a murder suicide with little evidence the shooter had any intent on shooting anyone else other than himself.

Faris was born before there was very much knowledge of the damage caused by alcohol. There is over a 50% chance he was prenatally exposed to alcohol using the statistics of drinking habits of women in their childbearing years.

Not Enough Info   Pre-1994   Fatal (and suicide)   <16

7. Nicholas Elliott, 16, Virginia Beach, Va., Dec. 16, 1988.

Nicholas Elliot, after reportedly being subjected to racial harassment, entered the Atlantic Shores Christian School, in Virginia Beach, Virginia, carrying a semi-automatic handgun his uncle had purchased for him several days prior. He shot and killed one teacher, wounded a second, and shot several times at a third as she ran from him. Another teacher tackled him, saving many lives, as Elliot was prepared to continue shooting all 200 rounds and set off three firebombs he carried in his backpack.

He is described as disturbed by Wall Street Journal, Erik Larson in his book Lethal Passage. He is the only black male in the Secret

Service study of school shooters. There is over a 50% chance he was prenatally exposed to alcohol using the statistics of drinking habits of women in their childbearing years, as he was born prior to any significant knowledge of the dangers of drinking during a pregnancy. Although black women do not drink as consistently during their childbearing years, the research shows a higher level of binge drinking, which can be more harmful to the brain.

Not Enough Info   Pre-1994   Fatal   >16

8. Cordell "Cory" Robb, 15, Orange County, Calif., Oct. 5, 1989.

Little can be found on this shooting. The intent is different than other school shootings, as Robb took hostages in order to get his stepfather to come to the school so he could kill him. Robb shot a student who taunted him.

There is over a 50% chance he was prenatally exposed to alcohol using the statistics of drinking habits of women in their childbearing years.

Not Enough Info   Pre-1994   Non-Fatal   <16

9. Eric Houston, 20, Olivehurst, Calif., May 1, 1992.

Eric Houston returned to his former school, upset after losing a job, wanting to get revenge for failing to graduate. He killed three students and the teacher who had given him a failing grade which resulting in him not graduating. He injured thirteen students in the rampage.

News reports said Houston was known to be unhappy and moody. One former friend said he thought he was a failure. He was in "slow learner" classes. He did poorly in regular education classes. At his trial, medical experts testified he had mental illness problems.

His learning disabilities and moody behaviors put him at a high probability of FASD. His judgment was certainly impaired. There is over a 50% chance he was prenatally exposed to alcohol using the statistics of drinking habits of women in their childbearing years as he was born in 1972 when very little was know of the dangers of drinking alcohol when pregnant.

Fits Profile   Pre-1994   Fatal   Adult

10. John McMahan, 14, Napa, Calif., May 14, 1992.

Bullied by other boys, he opened fire with a .357 in first period science class, wounding two students who he felt had bullied him. He then went outside, where he fired into the bushes until teachers were able to talk him into giving himself up.

There is very little information available on this shooting, as it did not result in a fatality and the shooter was a juvenile. Based on statistics, due to the fact warning labels were not placed on alcohol until November 17, 1989, there is a 50% chance his mother prenatally exposed him to alcohol.

Not Enough Info   Pre-1994   Non-Fatal   <16

11. Wayne Lo, 18, Great Barrington, Mass., Dec. 14, 1992.

At an exclusive college-prep boarding school, Lo killed two people and wounded four others. School administrators knew he had received a package from an ammo company and had decided to let him keep it. A student tried to warn counselors.

He personally replied to my emailed request for information and stated his mother did not drink alcohol. He sent a handwritten response that was scanned to email on his website. He wrote:

Thank you for your message. No, my mother never drank alcohol at all. Certainly not during her pregnancy with me. I've had MRI exams after the shootings for my criminal trial and no brain anomalies appeared what so ever. You should read Goneboy *by Gregory Gibson. There are chapters detailing the psychological evaluations I've received from both psychiatrists and psychologists. Perhaps that will offer you more insight for your study. Don't hesitate to ask me any questions you may have. I'll be glad to help.*
Wayne

Does not Fit Profile   Pre-1994   Fatal   College

12. Scott Pennington, 17, Grayson, Ky., Jan. 18, 1993.

Pennington entered East Carter High School, went to his high school English class, and killed Deanna McDavid. He then shot the janitor, Marvin Hicks, who attempted to intervene, and then held the class hostage.

Pennington was an honor student with a poor socioeconomic background. He had done a book report on a Stephen King novel where a student shot his teacher in front of the class and he wrote in his journal a veiled threat "They don't give out awards for what I have planned".

He was known as a "loner" and a "nerd" background and was teased because he wore glasses.

Not Enough Info   Pre-1994   Fatal   >16

13. Leonard McDowell, 21, Wauwatosa, Wis., Dec. 1, 1993.

Former student killed an associate principal who had handled his long history of disciplinary problems.

Fits Profile   Pre-   Fatal   Adult

14. Clay Shrout, 17, Union, Ky., May 26, 1994.

Clay Shrout killed four members of his family, and then walked into his trigonometry class five minutes late with his prom date following, flashed his gun and told the class he had had a bad day and he had just killed his family. The actions of Principal Stephen Sorrell and trigonometry teacher Carol Kanabroski helped save the lives of the 23 students held hostage. Sorrell called the room and asked a series of questions with yes or no answers, then had the teacher send someone out for as if there were a disciplinary reason. This allowed the principal to find out what was happening in the room. He eventually entered the room and convinced Shrout to give him the weapon.

Shrout has not been a model prisoner. In ten years, he had rung up 29 pages of disciplinary actions against him. He had avoided the death penalty by pleading guilty, but mentally ill for the murders of his parents and sisters.

Stout had an IQ of 160 according to published reports.   His actions were less of a school shooter and more of a mentally unstable son who acted against his family. Little is published regarding his behaviors prior to the incident.

Does not Fit Profile   Post 1994   Non-Fatal   >16

15. Nicholas Atkinson, 16, Greensboro, N.C., Oct. 12, 1994.

Suspended student shot and wounded assistant principal, killed himself.

Not Enough Info Pre-1994 Post 1994   Fatal (suicide)   >16 Suicide

178

16. Chad Welcher, 16, Manchester, Iowa, Nov. 8. 1994.

Fired two shotgun blasts into the principal's office, hitting a secretary.

Not Enough Info   Post 1994   Non-Fatal   Over 16

17. John Sirola, 13, Redlands, Calif., Jan. 23, 1995.

The principal at Sacred Heart School, a private Catholic school, reprimanded John Sirola, a Hispanic student. Sirola walked home, got his sawed-off shotgun, returned to school, shot and wounded the principal, then ran away. As he ran, he tripped and the gun went off, killing him. Authorities determined his motive was vengeance and the weapon was acquired from home. Sirola reportedly had problems with the dress code and authority.

Fits Profile   Post 1994   Fatal   < 16

18. Toby Sincino, 16, Blackville, S.C., Oct. 12, 1995.

Toby Sincino shot two teachers. He then shot himself in the head.

He was considered troubled, but he was also quiet and shy, friends said. He would brag about carrying a gun, but they didn't think he would ever use it. Toby got into trouble at school and with police. He occasionally picked on classmates but often felt he was the one being bullied.

Toby's aunt, Carolyn McCreary, said he had been undergoing counseling with the Department of Mental Health and was taking medicine for emotional problems. His medication, Zoloft, is frequently prescribed as an antidepressant. He was shuttled between the homes of estranged parents Randolph ``Pete'' Sincino and Gerlean McCreary Sincino.

Toby's academic career had declined steadily since the sixth grade, when Toby slapped a teacher. He was expelled from school in the 1994-95 school year but was allowed to return in 1995-96 on a strict probation. Then, he boasted to a friend that he had a gun. He was caught making an obscene gesture on a school bus the day before the shooting. He was suspended and would have been expelled because he was on probation.

Toby had a criminal record. Sources familiar with the case said Toby had an upcoming Family Court date on charges of pointing and presenting a firearm as well as simple assault. He had been sentenced to probation on prior Family Court charges of shoplifting and simple assault.

Every indicator is here for a high probability of prenatal exposure to alcohol. His behaviors, expulsions, low academics, diagnosis resulting in medication, estranged parents, boasting, disrupted school experience, trouble with the law all fit the profile of highly impacted FASD victim. The family situation, low socio-economic factor, and being shuttled between mother and father are red flags for alcohol abuse by the parents.

Fits Profile   Post 1994   Fatal (+ suicide)   >16

19. Jamie Rouse, 17, Lynnville, Tenn., Nov. 15, 1995.

Jaime Rouse had a history of problems in the small Tennessee school. He threatened other students and, at one time, scratched an upside down cross symbol into his forehead. He held his brother at gunpoint at one time, threatening to kill him. His parents took his gun away for a period of time. Upset over failing grade, he had a friend drive him to school, walked into the school carrying his Viper .22, walked up to two teachers talking in the hall and fired his gun at the teachers, killing one, wounding another. When firing at a third teacher, he hit a female student, who died.

The year before the shooting, he got into a violent fight with two other boys. When the teachers tried to break it up, he was totally out of control and would not calm down. He kept saying, "I will kill you." He was charged in that fight and suspended from school.

His father was a truck driver and his mother worked at home for a parts company. His father testified in court to being a hard drinking alcoholic and later in life, heavy into drugs. There is no testimony regarding his mothers drinking habits. His parents did not go to church, and as such, did not have a moral restraint from drinking. After all the children had been born and were attending school, his mother started putting pressure on his father to quit drinking. Research indicates a very high probability of his mother drinking due to the influence of her husband.

Fits Profile   Post 1994   Fatal   >16

20. Barry Loukaitis, 14, Moses Lake, Wash., Feb. 2, 1996.

Barry Loukaitis had one victim in mind when he opened the door to his algebra teacher, the student who, according to him and others, had been bullying him. He shot his algebra teacher who died immediately, and then killed two students, one being the boy he targeted.

He took the other students in the room hostage, but released the wounded. A physical education teacher, Jon Lane, came into the room to assist with removing the wounded. Lane tackled Loukaitis and held him until police arrived.

Loukaitis testified he had "mood swings." A classmate claimed that Loukaitis had thought it would be "fun" to go on a killing spree. It was reported he was on Ritalin at the time of the shooting. His mother told the jury her family had a history of depressive illness, which stretched back for four generations. Terry Loukaitis, Barry's father, said he was burdened with three generations' worth of depressive illnesses in his family. His mother also told the jury that she told her son of her plans to kill herself in front of her ex-husband and his new girlfriend on Valentine's Day, 1996. She said her son tried to encourage her not to do it and to channel her energies into writing about it.

A mother of one of the victims said, "He was mentally and emotionally ill and filled with rage. His needs went unmet, his cries for help ignored and his threats dismissed." -

While other organic causes may be in play, depression is a secondary disability of the brain damage of FASD. His age places his birth prior to the FDA warning labels on alcohol. His mother's state of depression puts her at risk for alcoholic behavior. Based on his mother's risk factors, his behaviors, his depression, the prescription of Ritalin, and his actions, there is a high probability he was prenatally exposed to alcohol.

Fits Profile   Post 1994   Fatal   <16

21 Anthony Gene Rutherford, 18; Patterson, Mo., March 25, 1996
Fits Profile   Post 1994   Fatal   >16

22. Jonathan Dean Moore, 15; Patterson, Mo., March 25, 1996
Fits Profile   Post 1994   Fatal   <16

23. Joseph Stanley Burris, 15; Patterson, Mo., March 25, 1996.
Fits Profile   Post 1994   Fatal   <16

The three students killed another student at a rural Christian school for troubled youths. They thought he might intervene in an attack they planned on the school. Mountain Park Baptist Church and Boarding School was a school for troubled students. Joseph Stanley Burris and Jonathan Dean Moore, both 15-years-old, Will Futrelle, 16, and Anthony Gene Rutherford, 18, planned to take over the school. A couple of days before the foursome was to set their plan in motion, Will "found God." Joseph, Jonathan and Anthony feared Will would reveal their plans to the staff. They led Will out in to the woods to "basically beat the crap out of him." However, the three were too aggressive and bludgeoned Will to death. The trio then tried to carry out their plan in a hurry, before they were caught. The trio tried to get into several of the staff homes to find weapons in order to hold the staff hostage until the news media arrived. However, they found no weapons and gave themselves up.

The fact these boys were placed in a school for troubled students places all three perpetrators into a very high probability for prenatal exposure to alcohol. Placement are typically due to behavior problems, academic problems, and trouble with the law, all secondary disabilities of FASD.

24. David Dubose Jr., 16, Scottsdale, Ga., Sept. 25, 1996.

A student at the DeKalb Alternative School for less than a week, Dubose shot and killed a teacher. The DeKalb Alternative School serves 4th through 12th grade students who have been expelled from their home schools.

The fact that David Dubose was expelled from the mainstream school and placed in an alternative school places him into a high probability for prenatal exposure to alcohol. Placement are typically due to behavior problems, academic problems, and trouble with the law, all secondary disabilities of FASD.

Fits Profile   Post 1994   Fatal   >16

25. Evan Ramsey, 16, Bethel, Alaska, Feb. 19, 1997.

Evan Ramsey told his friends he was going to bring a gun to school. The balcony was packed with onlookers who were waiting for the action. He killed a popular student and athlete Josh Palacios, 15, and then shot the principal, Ron Edwards, killing him. He wounded two others.

When Evan was 7, his father went to prison. His mother was an alcoholic, and he and his brothers were shipped off to a series of 11 different foster homes. In one of those homes, he suffered sexual abuse and humiliation, according to court testimony. He was depressed and attempted suicide at 10 years of age. By 10 years of age, Evan was using marijuana, getting poor grades and struggling to control an explosive temper.

He told researchers some kids had draped him with toilet paper and spit on his head, along with constantly calling him names. They also made fun of his grades, calling him brain-dead and retarded. A friend of Evan's recalled kids calling Ramsey 'spaz' and other degrading names,"

Without a doubt, Evan Ramsey is a victim of prenatal exposure to alcohol and his behaviors fit the profile of significant brain damage of FASD. The names he was called most likely were a result of his academic struggles and his violent outbursts of temper, thus the nickname "Spaz".

This is the first school shooter where the mother and father's drinking habits were part of the story. Not surprisingly, the drinking habits fit the stereotypical view of the mainstream press, as Ramsey is Native American. The only other shooter where the mother's drinking habits became part of the story was the Red Lake shooting, another Native American student. This obvious bias does nothing to help find the link between mothers drinking and school shooters.

Fits Profile   Post 1994   Fatal >16 Confirmed alcoholism of mother

26. Luke Woodham, 16, Pearl, Miss., Oct. 1, 1997.

Woodham stabbed and bludgeoned his mother to death at home then went to Pearl High School where he shot and killed two students and wounded seven other students. The motive was vengeance against his ex-girlfriend for breaking up with him, and against fellow students for picking on him. He was an honors student from a middle class family and his parents were divorced.

Prior to the incident he tortured and killed his dog by beating it with a club, stuffed it in a garbage bag, set it on fire, and threw it in a pond.

He had, reportedly, been teased since kindergarten. Students teased him constantly for being overweight and a nerd and taunted him using the words gay or fag. Even his mother called him fat, stupid, and lazy. Other boys bullied him routinely and, according to one fellow student, he "never fought back when other boys called him names"

Woodham wrote of torturing and killing his beloved dog, Sparkle. Woodham described how he and an accomplice beat his dog, then set it on fire and threw it in a pond. "I'll never forget the sound of her breaking under my might. I hit her so hard I knocked the fur off her neck . . . it was true beauty," he wrote.

Woodham testified about the murder of his mother and how he was influenced by one of the members of the small cult of fellow disgruntled students. He told of getting a knife and a pillow and walking to his mother's room. He said he could hear the cult leader's voice in his head throughout the process. "I just closed my eyes and fought with myself because I didn't want to do any of it. When I opened my eyes, my mother was lying in her bed."

All three psychologists who examined him prior to his trial agreed he had problems--narcissistic traits (which include, clinically speaking, lack of empathy and hypersensitivity to insult) and erratic coping skills. The psychologist for the defense testified he believed Woodham suffered from a serious depressive disorder.

Woodham did not have a good opinion of his mother. "She always told me that I wouldn't amount to anything," Woodham said. "She always told me that I was fat and stupid and lazy." His 24-year-old brother, he said, "used to pick on me--beat on me--when I was little." His parents' marriage ended in a bitter divorce. "She always never loved me." According Woodham, his mother blamed him for her divorce and problems with his brother. She spent many nights away from home.

Woodham also stated, "She said I was the reason my father left. She said I wouldn't amount to anything. She told me I was fat, stupid, and lazy. She was always against me."

Deborah Skipper, Metro Editor of the Clarion-Ledger in nearby Jackson, Mississippi wrote in 1998, "The only aspect of the story that remains not fully told is that of Mary Woodham. Who was she? In the telling of this story, she became a footnote: " Her family did not and does not want to talk about her. Luke Woodham's father remained an enigma and is unreachable. And so Mary Woodham disappeared into a journalistic footnote as the cell doors closed for life on her son."

While his mother was not able to defend herself against the accusations of Woodham, the divorced father and brother was not willing to speak at all to defend either Woodham or his mother. Her actions, the shaming and blaming language she used towards her son, and being away many nights suggest there were more problems than people were willing to address. Research shows a pregnant woman who does not want the pregnancy has a very high risk of drinking during the pregnancy.

Fits Profile   Post 1994   Fatal   >16

27. Michael Carneal, 14, West Paducah, Ky., Dec. 1, 1997.

Michael Carneal, the son of a prominent attorney, used stolen guns to kill three students and wound five in a prayer group holding their morning prayer in the common area of the school. One of the victims was someone he considered to be his ex-girlfriend. He was described as " shy and frail" standing barely 5 feet tall, weighing 110 pounds.

He wore thick glasses and played in the high school band. He felt alienated, pushed round, and picked on. Boys stole his lunch and constantly teased him. In middle school, someone pulled down his pants in front of his classmates. He was very hypersensitive. He later said he was so afraid that others would see him naked he covered the air vents in the bathroom. The school student gossip sheet published a statement that called him a "gay." He was devastated when students called him a "faggot."

Prior to the shooting, he stole two shotguns, two semiautomatic rifles, a pistol, and 700 rounds of ammunition. He spent the weekend showing them off to his classmates, then brought them to school hoping that they would bring him some respect from his tormentors. "I just wanted the guys to think I was cool," he said. When the cool guys ignored him, he began firing on a morning prayer circle, killing three classmates and wounding five others.

"He acted just like he had been caught with some minor offense." The principal said. "They saw him as a jokester," a local reverend said. "Even when he pulled the gun, they thought it was a toy. They had no idea he was capable of any of this."

Carneal was short, emotionally immature and was sometimes picked on by the older football players. It has been reported he was taking the prescription drug Ritalin. An examination of Mike's school essays and short stories showed that he felt weak and was constantly teased and picked on. "He's a very intelligent young man," the principal said. "He had some minor problems, but he's never been suspended from school."

Carneal had called his mother a bitch among other things in front of his friend on a trip with the family. He was downloading porn on the computer and selling it at school. He stole his father's pistol and used it to impress kids at school well before the shooting. He said, "Took gun to school in backpack the next day.(after he stole it from his dad's gun case) Felt powerful with it, like nobody would pick on him with it." and then sold it for $100 to a kid who was threatening to turn him in.

Michael reportedly was fixated on a girl he eventually killed. He called her nearly every night in the two months before the shootings, her mother says. Although he considered her his girlfriend, she considered him "a nuisance," and was only befriending him to help him.

Carneal had talked with friends about shooting students for over a year. Understandably, no one took him seriously. He told an investigator in the week before the shooting he had pulled a pistol on a couple of boys who had threatened to beat him up and the boys taunted him by saying, "You couldn't hurt anybody with that."

The local sheriff stated, "I've had no proof of any type of cult or atheists. I've heard just rumors of everything and I've seen no proof of any of that," he said. "All I've seen is a 14-year-old disturbed boy." Knives from the kitchen were discovered under his mattress after the shooting.

Carneal's family was Lutheran and attended the St. Paul Lutheran Church. His mother has a degree in English.

His behaviors fit the profile of a brain damaged by prenatal exposure to alcohol. After the shooting, he was diagnosed with Schizotypal Personality Disorder. Prior to the shooting, he was reportedly on Ritalin. His physical stature could be an indicator of prenatal exposure to alcohol, being described as short and frail. His family was Lutheran, a denomination that does not place a moral judgment on drinking alcohol. The research shows a high risk of prenatal exposure to alcohol for women who have a high social status, which would be a factor in this instance. His mother has a college degree, which is another high risk factor for women.

Fits Profile   Post 1994   Fatal   <16

28. Joseph "Colt" Todd, 14, Stamps, Ark., Dec. 15, 1997.

Todd shot two students in a non-fatal shooting. Two Stamps High School students were shot in the hip while waiting for school to begin. He was arrested in the nonfatal shootings four days later. Police say Todd shot the students from the perimeter of the school grounds. According to police, Todd complained he was tired of being picked on at school. He told police he wasn't targeting the two who were shot.

Not Enough Info   Post 1994   Non-Fatal   <16

29. Mitchell Johnson, 13, Jonesboro, Ark., March 24, 1998

Mitchell Johnson and Andrew Golden concocted a plan to shoot up their school. On March 24, Andrew Golden pulled the fire alarm and sent a shiver throughout our nation when he and Mitchell Johnson became the youngest boys charged with murder in the nation. They opened fire on the students and teachers as they filed out of the building for the fire alarm. Five were killed and 10 wounded. Johnson's mother had a confirmed pattern of drinking when she was young. She was pregnant when she married. The marriage did not last long. Reports indicate negligence on the part of both parents. Mitchell was involved in sexually deviant acts.

Fits Profile   Post 1994   Fatal   <16

30. Andrew Golden, 11, Jonesboro, Ark., March 24, 1998

There is little to find about Andrew. He was the younger participant in the massacre. He had a mean streak, according to some, and once killed a playmate's cat and dumped it in a trashcan. He also shot a classmate in the face with a pellet gun. Friends and neighbors described Andrew Golden as evil, demented, "a troublemaker," and "always threatening people."

Because of his age, little was given about his academics and school related behaviors. He spent most of his time with his grandparents. His father was a truck driver and his mother worked at the post office. He reportedly, was on Ritalin.

Fits Profile   Post 1994   Fatal   <16

31. Andrew Wurst, 14, Edinboro, Pa., April 25, 1998.

Andrew killed a teacher and wounded three students at a dinner-dance. He had talked of killing people and taking his own life. A psychologist concluded in his official report that Andrew suffers from "a major mental illness, with psychotic thinking and delusions of persecution and grandeur" and is in need of long-term inpatient treatment with medication.

Andrew was average in size at 5'8" and 125 lbs. He was not particularly athletic. Andrew was not under a doctor's treatment and did not take any medications. He struggled academically, with his grades slipping year by year until he was getting mostly Ds and Fs in eighth grade.

He frequently drank whiskey or vodka with orange juice, getting a "buzz," but not drunk. In eighth grade, he began to use marijuana occasionally, which he said made his body go numb. Several classmates told police that Andrew had bragged constantly about his drug use in recent months. He began having suicidal ideas when he was 10. His family attended St. George Catholic Church.

Fits Profile   Post 1994   Fatal   <16

32. Jacob Davis, 18, Fayetteville, Tenn., May 19, 1998.

An honor student three days before graduation, Davis used a rifle to shoot another boy in a dispute over a girl. Looking back, Davis says he was secretly troubled as a kid, even though he seemed normal to others: "Most of the people I would say that knew me refused to believe it. It just didn't make sense." He lived with his stepmother.

Not Enough Information   Post 1994   Fatal   >16

33. Kip Kinkel, 15, Springfield, Ore., May 21, 1998.

After being expelled for bringing a gun to school, Kinkel killed his parents, then killed two students in the cafeteria. He wounded 25.

Kip Kinkel had a difficult school career. He was held back in first grade because Kip's parents and teachers felt he lacked maturity and had slow emotional and physical development. His parents asked that he be tested for learning disabilities in second grade. He screened average in his neurological test, but had a low score in his motor skills and had difficulty with spelling, even his last name and had an abnormally high level of frustration and anxiety. He was retested in third grade for Special Education services and qualified. He was diagnosed with a learning disability in fourth grade. By all accounts, he was hyperactive, rebellious, stubborn, and a poor student who preferred to act as the class clown rather than bear down on his studies.

By seventh grade, he was hanging out with friends who made his mother nervous. For a while, he was prescribed Ritalin. He had a fixation on building bombs. In eighth grade, he was caught shoplifting and bought an old sawed off shotgun from a friend and hid it from his parents. While on a snowboarding trip, he and a friend were arrested for throwing rocks off an overpass onto the passing cars. He was describes as having a violent temper and was quick to lash out at anyone who crossed him.

Following the Bend incident, Kip's mother brought Kip to see psychologist Jeffrey Hicks. According to Dr. Hicks, his mother was worried about Kip. She told Dr. Hicks about brushes with the law. She told him she was worried about his temper and his "extreme interest in guns, knives, and explosives," and was afraid he could harm himself or others. Testimony in court revealed Kip had a strained relationship with his father. In his notes, Hicks wrote "Kip became tearful when discussing his relationship with his father. He reported that Kip thought his mother viewed him as 'a good kid with some bad habits' while his father saw him as 'a bad kid with bad habits.' He felt his father expected the worst from him." He often bragged about torturing and killing animals.

Dr. Hicks diagnosed Kip with Major Depressive Disorder and concluded "Kip had difficulty with learning in school, had difficulty managing anger, some angry acting out and depression."

Kip was suspended for two days for kicking another student in the head after the student shoved him. Kip was angry that the other boy did not get punished. Soon after, Kip got a three-day suspension for throwing a pencil at another boy. Shortly after this incident, which his mother felt the school was overreacting, he was prescribed 20 milligrams of Prozac per day. He took the Prozac for three months.

His dad purchased a pistol for him, but kept it under lock and key. He later bought another pistol from a friend, but kept it hidden from his parents. His dad then bought him a .22 rifle.

Kinkel's dad was concerned because Kip had started hanging out with a tougher group of kids, playing with explosives, and that he was becoming difficult to manage, more secretive and was having troubles in school. A friend of Kip's sister, Kristen said, "They tried to discipline him, and they tried to keep him from making more bombs," she said. "But at some point, Kristin said, they just pretty much had given up on being able to control him." (CNN News)

On May 20, Kip was arrested for having a handgun in his locker. He had made arrangements to buy the handgun from another student, who stole the gun from his father. He was handcuffed and taken from the school and suspended pending expulsion. His father picked him up from the police station and brought him home.

Later that afternoon, Kip killed his father in the kitchen with one shot to the head from behind. When his friends called, he told them his father was not home, but was at the bar. When his mother came home, he shot her six times.

After sleeping in the house where his dead parents lay, the next morning he left for school with his guns. He entered the school and started shooting. Before five other students could wrestle him to the ground, two students were dead and 25 were wounded. He left behind a booby-trapped bedroom at home.

In his book, *Base Instincts*, (MetroBooks, 2001) Dr. Jonathan Pincus writes about his examination of Kinkel. He states Kinkel was subjected to verbal abuse from his parents. He also determined Kinkel's physical examination and brain scan showed abnormalities.
Fits Profile   Post 1994   Fatal   <16

34. Shawn Cooper, 16, Notus, Idaho, April 16, 1999.
Shawn rode the bus to school with a shotgun wrapped in a blanket. He pointed the gun at a secretary and students, and then shot twice into a door and at the floor. He had a death list, but told

one girl he wouldn't hurt anyone. He surrendered. Cooper had been taking Ritalin when he fired the shotgun's rounds and was reported to be on a mix of antidepressants.

There is not enough information to determine FASD status, but it cannot be ruled out, especially due to the mix of medication.

Not Enough Info   Post 1994   Non-Fatal   <16

35. Eric Harris, 17, Columbine, Colo., April 20, 1999.

Harris and Klebold killed 12 students and one teacher, wounded 23 students, and then committed suicide.

This tragedy has been analyzed more than any other. The one question that has not been asked is whether the mothers of the two killers drank any alcohol when pregnant. Here are some reported behaviors, physical features, and facts that give cause to ask the question.

Eric Harris

Harris' father was a military man. He was an Air Force pilot, a job that is notorious for the drinking that happens. He and Katherine had a church wedding at First Presbyterian in Englewood on April 17, 1970. This was well before the public awareness of the dangers of drinking during pregnancies and Eric was born seven years before warnings were placed on all alcohol. Katherine Harris stayed home when Kevin and Eric were young; keeping busy with military-wives luncheons, volunteer projects and school functions.

The facts that they were Presbyterian, a denomination that does not require abstinence from alcohol, they were young parents in a high risk, high stress occupation, moving often, and the fact Wayne Harris, Eric's dad was quoted in his 20th year reunion as writing: "What I like? Eating, drinking, flying and loving, not necessarily in that order" would put them at a very high probability of Katherine Harris prenatally exposing Eric to alcohol.

Eric displayed at least one physical characteristic that is evidenced in 7% of FASD victims, a concave chest. This physical feature caused teasing from his peers. He did not want to remove his T-shirt in gym class. He also was undersized, standing 5'61/2" tall, 135-140 lbs. He was shorter than his brother.

Eric started getting into trouble by all reports when he was in high school. He displayed his violent temper, to the mother of a friend. One day a former friend was driving by the bus stop near his house. Eric threw a chunk of ice, breaking his windshield. This former friend, Brooks told his mother, who immediately drove to the bus stop and confronted Eric. She got his backpack and told him she was going to talk to his mother. He grabbed onto her car, screaming, his face turning red. She later stated he reminded her of an animal attacking a vehicle at a wild-animal park.

Judy Brown recalled Wayne Harris calling the Browns. "He said his son was afraid of me and that's why he was hanging on the door handle", Judy Brown said. "I said 'Your son's not afraid. Your son is terrifying. Your son is violent.'"

According to court papers the sheriff's office had been aware them that Eric Harris had threatened to kill another student back in 1998. After being arrested for theft, Harris was remanded to a juvenile diversion project in Jefferson County. In documents filled out in his diversion program, Harris' own words in some of the diversion documents state, for example: "Short temper, often get angry at almost anything I don't like, like people I have no respect for trying to tell me what to do. People telling me what to think. I have too many inside jokes or thoughts to have very many friends. I hate too many things."

Harris also noted he experienced anger, anxiety, depression, disorganized thoughts, homicidal thoughts, jealousy, loneliness, mood swings, obsessive thoughts, racing thoughts, stress, suspiciousness, and a temper.

Eric Harris was diagnosed with a psychiatric problem that needed medication. He began taking an antidepressant called Luvox. When he tried to enlist in the Marine Corps in early April, he said did not tell the truth about his medication and was rejected.

One of the reasons the behaviors did not present themselves earlier in life was the highly structured home setting. Research shows FASD brains are most successful in high structure. As he got older, the structure lessened and the behaviors became more evident, in my opinion, culminating in the staggering loss of life at Columbine.

    Fits Profile   **Post 1994**   **Fatal(+suicide)**   **>16**

36. Dylan Klebold, 18, Columbine, Colo., April 20, 1999

Many see Eric Harris as the leader of the two. He authored the journal with the description of the plot. His website was filled with threats. He was the vocal one of the pair, with Dylan seen as a shy outcast.

When the two were arrested for theft, Dylan was the first to confess and then Eric told the investigators the theft was Dylan's idea.

His mother was raised Jewish and converted to Christianity when she married his father. They attended a Lutheran church, a denomination that condones drinking alcohol. A poster was reportedly hanging in Dylan's room that showed how to make "shooters". He preferred to be called by the name "Vodka." This shows a liberal view towards the drinking of alcohol, which would place his mother in the 50-60% of mothers who were drinking during their childbearing years.

Dylan is one of the 4 school shooters of the Secret Services study that does not fit the profile for FASD, although prenatal exposure to alcohol cannot be ruled out.
Does not Fit Profile   Post 1994 (+suicide)   >16

37. Thomas Solomon, 15, Conyers, Ga., May 20, 1999.

Thomas Solomon was distraught over being dumped by his girlfriend. He turned sullen and talked of bringing a gun to school. He was described as a quiet kid with a few close friends. He brought two guns to school and started firing indiscriminately at students, wounding six. His family moved to Conyers two years prior to the shooting and he lived with his mother, stepfather and 13 year-old sister. T.J., as he was called, was taking Ritalin, which is usually prescribed for hyperactivity. A friend of the family said that his grades had been falling during the past year and that he had been medically treated for depression. He was also a Boy Scout and attended Catholic Church.

The fact he was prescribed Ritalin and his family attended the Catholic Church, a church that condones drinking alcohol, fits the profile of prenatal exposure to alcohol.
Fits Profile   Post 1994   Non-Fatal   <16

38. Victor Cordova Jr., 12, Deming, N.M., Nov. 19, 1999.

Victor, a student who lived in Mexico and went to school in New Mexico brought a gun to school and shot a student in the head, killing her. He had a history of emotional problems and was sometimes violent. He had been dealing with depression, a violent temper and the loss of his 31-year-old mother who died of cancer six months earlier. "He acts like he's fine, but when he's in another place, he acts like a bear. He's bad," said Cordova Jr.'s sister, 10-year-old Karen . "He's always sad, he doesn't want to talk. He's always violent. He'd yell and throw things." He had talked about committing suicide a month after his mother died. "But Victor (Jr.) said it was a joke," Sonia Cordova said. The boy's father said the boy had been prescribed medication for his temperament two years ago by a Ciudad Juarez doctor, but that the boy stopped taking it after a short while because he grew more depressed.

Fits Profile   Post 1994   Fatal   <16

39. Seth Trickey, 13, Fort Gibson, Okla., Dec. 6, 1999.

Because there was not a fatality at this shooting, little information could be found. Trickey brought a gun to school and wounded four students outside Fort Gibson Middle School.

Reports indicate Seth was receiving treatment from a psychologist for 9 months prior to the shooting. He was on prescription medication and had been given a dose of steroids three weeks prior to the shooting for treatment of poison ivy. His parents attended First United Methodist Church, a denomination that does not condemn drinking.

There is not enough information to determine FASD status, but it cannot be ruled out, especially due to the mix of medication and the fact his mother attended a church that did not condemn drinking.

Not Enough Info   Post 1994   Non-Fatal   <16

40. Nathaniel Brazill, 13, Lake Worth, Fla., May 26, 2000.

Nathaniel had been sent home for throwing water balloons on the last day of school. He returned with a gun and killed a teacher. Nathaniel Brazill is the son of Nathaniel Brazill Sr., 42, a postal worker, and Polly Ann Powell, 35, a cook at a local retirement home. They did not marry. His mother, Polly, was involved in several abusive relationships. Police reported that there were 17 domestic incident reports at her home in the six years prior to the shooting. Powell has been married twice. She says that she divorced her first husband because he was abusive.

One of Ms. Powell's partners demanded that Nathaniel move out of the house. Mother said and like any other kid he was impulsive, eager to impress friends, ignorant of the long-term consequences of things he does. A teacher said he was increasingly showing anger. His grades were dropping in 6th grade.

Fits Profile   Post 1994   Fatal   <16

Additional Shooter List

1. Roger Needham, 17, Lansing, MI, Feb. 22, 1978

Roger Needham brought a pistol to school. He shot and killed one student and injured a second. Both were students who teased Needham and tried to get him to fight.

According to classmates he fidgeted a lot, not enough to cause trouble, just enough to be a distraction. His teachers found him a disappointment academically. Classmates found him an out-and-out weirdo. There were rumors around campus that he talked about building atomic weapons, burning down houses and throwing bombs in school.

His father, a single parent with three kids, was raising him. His father's passions were guns, World War II and Adolf Hitler's Nazi regime.

Tests conducted after the shooting put Needham's IQ in the genius range. "He is highly intelligent, hostile, intensely angry at everyone," psychiatrist Ames Robey wrote in a report to prosecutors. Roger had just turned 5 when his parents divorced. The judge found truth to allegations that the elder Needham had been "guilty of extreme and repeated cruelty" toward his wife. She was awarded custody of Roger and his younger sister and brother. Five years later, the judge transferred custody of all three children to Needham. His mother resettled in the Pacific Northwest, where she said she was communicating with the boy by ESP.

Does not fit Profile   Pre 1994   Fatal   <16

2. Ricky Lopez, 13, April 1977, Whitharral, TX

Ricky Lopez fatally shot Mr. Tripp, the school principal, because "the devil told him to." He pleaded insanity at his trial. He was placed in a state institute and released after his 18th birthday.

Not Enough Information   Pre 1994   Fatal   <16

3. Brenda Ann Spencer, 16, January 29, 1979, San Diego, CA.

On 29 January 1979, 16-year-old Brenda Ann Spencer opened fire on children arriving at Cleveland Elementary School in San Diego from her house across the street, killing two men and wounding eight students and a police officer.

Her mother and father divorced when she was about nine years old. She was living with her father. As to what impelled her into this form of murderous madness, she told a reporter, "I don't like Mondays. This livens up the day."

According to a report written by the police negotiators who spoke with her during the six-hour standoff, she made such comments to them as "There was no reason for it, and it was just a lot of fun"; "It was just like shooting ducks in a pond"; and the kids "looked like a herd of cows standing around, it was really easy pickings."

Spencer pled guilty to two counts of murder and assault with a deadly weapon and was sentenced to 25 years to life in prison.

Fits Profile   Pre 1994   Fatal   <16

4. James Wilson, 19, Greenwood, SC, September 6, 1988

James Wilson, 19, opened fire in a Greenwood, S.C. elementary school. He shot seven students and two teachers. Two 8-year-old girls died.

Wilson pleaded guilty but mentally ill and has been sentenced to death in South Carolina's electric chair. Wilson had been in and out of the hands of psychiatrists for years. Since the age of 14 he had been given psychiatric drugs, including Xanax, Valium, Thorazine and Haldol. He was withdrawing from Xanax at the time of the shooting spree. At nineteen, he was a dropout who never held a job.

Wilson acted as a result of an "irresistible impulse. Wilson's sister said that her parents "did not want" Wilson and sent him off to live with his grandparents. Wilson stood out as unusual among his peers for his "trance-like" or "zombie-type" appearance. He displayed violence and disrespect toward his parents, grandparents, or other authority figures. Wilson had shown obsessive-compulsive symptoms since he was 8 or 9. These included washing his hands compulsively, not allowing any of his sisters to touch the refrigerator door, refusing to drink out of anything but a Dixie cup, and only opening doors with a handkerchief.

Additionally, his psychologist testified that Wilson suffered borderline personality disorder and schizotypal personality disorder. She testified that Wilson's grandmother had described Wilson as getting worse over time, talking to himself and others who were not actually there, and becoming increasingly paranoid about other people being out to get him. Wilson made threats to his parents and to his grandparents." describe chronologically the gradual deterioration in his functioning from his early childhood through adolescence and the difficulty that he had in school. The court was presented evidence of substance abuse and mental illness in Wilson's extended family,

Fits Profile   Pre 1994   Fatal   >16

5. Tronneal Mangum, 13, January 27, 1997

Tronneal Magnum shot and killed another 13-year-old student, Jean Kamel, in front of their school. Both were students at Conniston and had numerous prior violent confrontations, including Mangum's kicking Jean Kamel in his prosthetic leg.

Mangum was suspended from school, tried as an adult and sentenced to life without parole. He had been suspended from school for a prior altercation with the same student over a watch.

Not Enough Information   Fatal   <16

6. Dedrick Owens, 6, Mount Morris Township, MI, Feb. 19, 2000

Dedrick Owens was only six-years-old when he shot six-year-old Kayla Rolland dead.

Even though he had only been present in the school for two weeks or so before he shot his classmate dead, he had already built up a reputation as a bully. He had stabbed another pupil.

His father was incarcerated in the County jail. He told the sheriff his son aggressively towards the other children because "he hated them."

When Owens pushed one of his classmates, she pushed back and he fell over. Swearing to get even with the girl who had humiliated him, he went home, got a .32 automatic from the crack house where he was living, and returned to confront her.

He shot Kayla in the chest at point-blank range. He had just pointed the pistol at another little girl and said, "I hate you".

Owens and his brother had been staying with their mother's brother after she had been evicted from her home. One local newspaper described the place where Owens had found the gun thus:

"The ramshackle house is surrounded by mud-caked trash, and the front yard is cluttered with an empty vodka bottle and a rusting black Camaro."

He was too young to be prosecuted.

Fits Profile   Fatal   <16

7. Charles "Andy" Williams, 15, Santee, CA, March 5 2001

Williams killed two fellow students and wounded 13 others at Santana High School in Santee, California, in San Diego County.

Williams was born to Charles Jeffery and Linda Williams. He was born about 2 weeks premature. His mother worked for the US Army. Williams lived the first 8 months of his life with his mother, but seldom saw her after that. In 1990, the couple divorced. Williams went to live with his father, and his brother went to live with their mother.

After moving to Santee, California from Twentynine Palms, Williams felt he was targeted for physical and emotional bullying in school. In an attempt to fit in, he began to spend time with a crowd of skateboarders. Williams was accepted within this peer group; however, at times, these individuals also teased or picked on him. In February 2001, just before his 15th birthday, Williams received news that one of his best friends from Twentynine Palms was killed in a bus accident. Williams was sentenced to 50 years to life in prison.

Fit Profile   Fatal   <16   Post-Secret Service

8. Elizabeth Catherine Bush, 14, Williamsport, PA, March 7, 2001

Bush wounded student Kimberly Marchese in the cafeteria of Bishop Neumann High School. She was reportedly depressed and frequently teased. Marchese described Bush as a disturbed girl who had emotional and family problems. She was taking Prozac at the time of the shooting.

Before attending the Roman Catholic school, Bush had attended public school in the Jersey Shore Area School District. When she went there, classmates on the school bus would call her a homosexual and other names or even throw stones at her after school, her mother said. Problems persisted at the new school.

Fits Profile   Non-Fatal   <16   Post-Secret Service

9. Jason Hoffman, 18, Granite Hills, CA., March 22, 2001

Jason Hoffman opened fire on the principal and vice principals' offices from the outside. Five people were either injured by shrapnel or suffered severe symptoms from the traumatic experience but no victims incurred bullet wounds. A policeman shot and wounded Hoffman. He had been diagnosed as clinically depressed and had been prescribed Celexa and Effexor. He hung himself in jail.

According to court records, his father was alcoholic and once spent time in jail on a child-endangerment charge. His parents never married. They lived together until they separated in 1983. His mother said she moved out of Hoffman's house in 1983, when she said he threw the boy, then 3 months old, across the room at her.

Classmates have described him as quiet, moody and prone to angry outbursts. Handwritten notes revealed he thought the Dean of the school was somehow to blame for his failure to get into the Navy. His dad said the boy was difficult to raise. "Any time Jason doesn't get his way, he throws a tantrum and I don't let him get away with it," his father stated. He also asked the court order the mother into parenting classes so she can learn to cope with the problems of raising this boy.

A student said she sat next to Hoffman and was afraid of him. She said he was hostile and rarely spoke. Once, for no apparent reason, he broke his pencil into little pieces in the middle of class.

"He would never talk except if he got really mad," she said.

"He was picked on because he was one of the scrawniest guys," another student said. "People called him 'freak,' 'dork,' 'nerd,' stuff like that."

Fits Profile   Fatal   >16   Post-Secret Service

10. Donald R. Burt, Jr., 17, Gary, Ind., March 30, 2001

One student was killed by Burt, who had been expelled from Lew Wallace High School. He had been expelled the previous school year and had withdrawn for the 2000-2001 school year. When Burt attended Lew Wallace, a Behavioral Assessment was completed, which stated that he exhibited aggressive behavior and had expressed homicidal ideations. Burt was eventually convicted for the murder of Neal.

Fits Profile   **Fatal**   **>16**   **Post-Secret Service**

11. Cory Baadsgaard, 16, Mattawa, WA April 10, 2001

Cory Baadsgaard took a rifle to his high school and took 23 classmates and a teacher hostage. According to another student, "Cory was yelling and then he just stopped, looked down at the gun in his hand and woke up." Fortunately, no one was hurt. Cory had been taking Effexor and had no memory of the incident.

Does Not Fit Profile   **non- Fatal**   **>16**   **Post-Secret Service**

12. Corey Ramos, 17, Springfield, Mass., December 5, 2001

Reverend Theodore Brown, principal of the school, caught 17-year-old Corey Ramos wearing a hooded jacket in the hallway between classes. Wearing the hood over the head is against Springfield's policy, a school for troubled teens. Theodore told Corey to remove the hood, but the boy ignored his principal. Theodore followed Corey into a classroom where the two argued. Ramos pulled out a knife and stabbed the principal several times in the chest and abdomen, killing him.

Fits Profile   **Fatal**   **>16**   **Stabbing**   **Post-Secret Service**

13. James Sheets, 14, Red Lion, PA, April 24, 2003

Sheets killed principal Eugene Segro of Red Lion Area Junior High School before killing himself. Some students said Sheets was troubled and had hinted that he planned to kill himself and Segro, but they could offer no reasons why. But many others who knew Sheets said the eruption of violence seemed completely out of character.

Sheets was a football and baseball player who sat at the "jock" table during pre-homeroom morning gatherings in the cafeteria. He was a hunter, like other members of his family, but seldom discussed the sport with his friends. He exhibited no fascination with guns. Sheets lived with his mother and stepfather

Police and Red Lion Area Superintendent Larry Macaluso said Sheets was not known as a troublemaker. They were unaware of any disputes between Sheets and Segro.

Some students, though, said that Sheets had recently been disciplined at school and that he also was upset by a breakup with a girlfriend.

Classmates and school officials described Sheets as a quiet teen, who was pleasant but not particularly popular or outgoing. He was an average student and not regarded a troublemaker.

Not Enough Information   Fatal   <16   Post-Secret Service

14. Jon Romano, 16, Greenbush, NY, February 9, 2004

Jon Romano opened fire with a shotgun hitting Special education teacher Michael Bennett in the leg. The boy was treated with medication for depression. Romano was an emotionally disturbed young man who was being treated for problems ranging from depression to anxiety. "He had a lot of problems," a law enforcement official said. "He had emotional problems." In recent years his behavior has been getting worse, and last spring he was not allowed to attend school, according to a school official. Instead, officials said, home schooling was provided.

Fits Profile   Non-Fatal   >16   Post-Secret Service

15. Jason Clinard, 14, Cumberland City, TN, March 2, 2005

Jason Clinard walked up to his bus stop as the bus doors opened, pulled a handgun from his jacket pocket and fired six shots at the bus driver, killing her. In court, the psychiatrist testified that the teen heard voices and suffered from major depression with psychotic features. He also diagnosed Clinard with recurring depressive disorder and intermittent explosive disorder, a condition in which the individual's anger causes them to act impulsively. At the time of the shooting, his father's health was deteriorating, his mother's work took excessive time away from home, and he had been through the recent death of a grandparent. In the year leading up to the shooting, two of Clinard's friends attempted suicide and his stepsister moved her family into his home. The psychiatrist suggested Clinard could possibly have brain damage, after suffering an unusually high number of childhood accidents, including being hit in the head with a baseball and a sledgehammer that resulted in broken bones and head injuries.

Clinard's facial features show characteristics of fetal alcohol syndrome.

Fits Profile   Fatal   >16   Post-Secret Service

16. Ken Bartley Jr., 14, Jacksboro, TN, Nov. 8, 2005

Bartley shot and killed an assistant principal at Campbell County High School and seriously wounded two other administrators. The boy had been in and out of trouble while in middle school and had spent about a year and a half in a residential juvenile treatment program. He had a reputation as a " bad kid."

He was on probation from earlier juvenile court woes that included drug use and a violent encounter with his mother.

"I've seen him getting scared before about getting into trouble," a friend said. "I could see him just panicking. He makes stupid mistakes. He's so immature."

In the early 1990's, his father killed a man and avoided trial when the killing was justified as self-defense.

Fits Profile   Fatal   >16   Post-Secret Service

17. Thomas White, 13, Joplin, MO, October 9, 2006

Thomas White fired a gun inside his middle school after confronting two others students and his principal. He was wearing a mask and had pointed the gun at the principal, the assistant superintendent and two students. After firing a shot into the ceiling and breaking a water pipe, his gun jammed. Police confronted him and took him into custody. The police found a note in his backpack stating he had placed an explosive in the school. No one was injured in the incident.

Thomas White hated school. He was failing four out of his six classes at Memorial Middle School. He had gotten into trouble at home and apparently did not see how he could get better grades. Thomas White told his interrogators "he just wanted to scare people," When asked specifically whom he was trying to scare, he'd told them "all the teachers," according to the brief. He was evaluated at the Western Missouri Mental Health Center in Kansas City by court order, and a psychiatric report was delivered to the court that deemed the boy mentally unfit to understand legal proceedings and to assist in his own defense.

Wright had been a special education student most of his academic life with limited ability to make good choices. He told fictitious stories about time he had spent in Oklahoma about his gang involvement with the "Playboy Gangsta Crips" and drive-by shootings. He was highly impulsive. He had a complete lack of remorse for his actions.

Fits Profile   Fatal   <16   Post-Secret Service

18. Douglas Chanthabouly, 18, Tacoma, Wash., Jan. 3, 2007

Chanthabouly pointed a handgun at his victim in the hallway of Henry Foss High School and fired a fatal shot into his face. He fired twice more, hitting him in the lower left side and left buttock.

He had a history of mental illness. He was admitted to a psychiatric hospital in Kirkland two years prior to the shooting after attempting suicide. He was confused at times, somewhat depressed and having hallucinations, a court ordered psychiatrist wrote in her evaluation. He "appears to have difficulty with concentration" and said he has trouble remembering things since he began suffering psychotic symptoms about two years ago, she wrote. His ongoing psychotic symptoms were reduced but not extinguished with medication.

Students at Foss who knew both students have speculated that the attack may have been gang related. While police have said repeatedly that the shooting wasn't gang related, friends and acquaintances of both youths believe otherwise. "I think its gang related -- just because of the kind of person Sam used to be," said his friend, speculating that the attack might have been retribution for a perceived offense from years ago.

Fits Profile   Fatal   >16   Post-Secret Service

19. David Turner, 17, Midland, Michigan, March 7, 2007

David Turner shot his girlfriend four times outside Herbert Henry Dow High School before killing himself in the parking lot. Turner and his girlfriend both attended an alternative high school in the area until March 5, when she transferred to H.H. Dow High. Authorities believe that Turner acted because she had broken off the relationship and transferred to Dow High to distance herself from him. Turner was previously convicted of stealing firearms, as well as a count of domestic abuse against his mother. He was sentenced to 18 months' probation in December 2006 with stipulation that he must not use a firearm. His girlfriend was four months pregnant with Turner's baby at the time of the shooting. He had a history of abrupt mood changes.

Fits Profile   Fatal   >16   Post-Secret Service

20. Chad Escobedo, 15, Gresham, OR, April 10. 2007

Chad Escobedo shot the windows out of two classrooms from outside Springwater Trail High School, injuring ten students with shrapnel and broken glass, two of which required stitches.   His motive was to shoot at classrooms because he was unhappy that an instructor had called his parents.   The classrooms he hit, however, were not his intended targets. Springwater Principal Larry Bentz said he knows Escobedo "quite well" and had been counseling Escobedo about troubles the teen was having at home.   Students said he sometimes lied about things.

Fits Profile   Fatal   >16   Post-Secret Service

21. Greg Wright, 17, Oroville, CA, September 28, 2007

A 17-year old student held three girls hostage at Las Plumas High School for nearly an hour after releasing twenty-seven other students and an instructor in a band room. The gunman allegedly fired numerous gunshots through the ceilings while the three girls were in his custody. When police arrived, the gunman peacefully surrendered.

In District Attorney Mike Ramsey's opinion, he's "a dangerous young man with a proclivity and fascination with guns and violence" with an extensive juvenile record from Oklahoma.   He was primed to kill someone that day, took a bunch of students hostage, fired off his gun and scared them to death.

Gregory was a sweet-natured but not very bright student.   He had been in special education most of his life.   He was reported to not be   mature enough to understand the consequences of his behaviors. He was impulsive.   He had never hurt anyone.

Fits Profile   Fatal   >16   Post-Secret Service

22. Asa Coon, 14, Cleveland Ohio, Oct. 10, 2007

Asa H. Coon shot and injured two students and two teachers before he killed himself. The victims' injuries were not life threatening. He was reportedly upset about a suspension so he went on a shooting spree in SuccessTech Academy. He committed suicide when police executed a manhunt search. Coon and another student were suspended after they apparently got in a fight outside the school the day previous to the shooting.

He had been diagnosed bipolar and was refusing medication. Coon had a previous arrest last year for a domestic violence incident, and police had been to his home before for incidents that involved weapons.

Students described the gunman as being "odd." Coon spent time in two juvenile facilities after a domestic violence episode and was given home detention, and he was suspended from school last year for trying to injure a student, according to juvenile court records. He had a history of mental health problems and threatened to commit suicide last year while in a mental health center.

Asa Coon grew up in a family where violence seemed commonplace. His older brother, Stephen, was twice charged with both domestic violence and assault by the time he was 13. He was recently released from prison.

According to court records, back in 1998, Asa was involved in a neglect case. The details are unclear but social workers say Asa who was around five at the time had burns on different parts of his body. Court records show that his father's whereabouts are largely unknown. When Asa was 3, his mother, Lori Looney, was investigated by social workers after they were alerted that she often left her four children with drug addicts. Courts in New York found the children were neglected.

"He was a very hyper kid," a neighbor said. "He constantly yelled at his mom or anybody else. He was pretty violent."

Fits Profile   Fatal   >16   Post-Secret Service

23. Brandon McInerney, 14, Silver Strand Beach, CA, Feb. 12, 2008

McInerney walked into a classroom and shot another student twice in the back of the head. In the days before the shooting, Brandon had been heard telling the victim, a gay student, to leave him alone, that he would hurt him. Brandon was arrested a few blocks from the school and later charged with first-degree murder and a hate crime. Three weeks after Brandon's 14th birthday, prosecutors announced he would be tried as an adult.

Brandon's childhood was marred by violence. Brandon was 6 when his parents separated, but problems between Kendra and William McInerney started before Brandon was born. Kendra McInerney, Brandon's mother, claimed a night of partying in 1993 ended in a fight and William shooting her in the elbow, breaking it in several places, according to court records. Still, they married later that year, and Brandon was born in January 1994. (This timeline clearly confirms prenatal exposure to alcohol.)

Brandon and his two older half-brothers often witnessed his parents fighting, according to court records. In 2000, his dad pleaded no contest to a domestic battery charge against his mother. He was sentenced to 10 days in jail and ordered to attend domestic violence classes. The couple separated in August 2000.

His mother claimed that in September 2000, his dad choked her "until she was almost unconscious" and dragged her by her hair during a fight about prescription drugs, according to court records. The medicine belonged to one of Brandon's half-brothers. Each parent claimed the other was taking the boy's pills.

He lived with his mother and half-brothers, or with his father a few miles away. Custody changed several times. Court documents included conditions that neither parent use drugs or alcohol when having custody of Brandon or required drug testing at either one's request.

His mother started using methamphetamine at age 20. His mother's house was considered a "drug house." Brandon would live most of the time with his dad and grandfather and stay with his mom on weekends.

Brandon would intimidate others. A parent of a classmate said her son has known Brandon since the second grade, and over the years she saw him alternately be charming and a bully "Brandon picked on what was different," she said. Other classmates remember seeing Brandon's sometimes-aggressive side.

Alcohol is a part of his family's problems. In 2002, his dad pleaded guilty to drunk driving and being an unlicensed driver. He served five days in jail and was fined.

Fits Profile   Fatal   <16   Post-Secret Service

24. Jamar B. Siler 15, Knoxville, TN, August 21, 2008

Siler shot and killed 15-year-old Ryan McDonald in the school cafeteria. He was charged with first-degree murder and an unspecified probation violation.

The public defender said his office has represented the boy in the past, but he didn't know the exact nature of the cases. Both Siler and McDonald had faced charges as juveniles.

Jamar Siler was adopted. His sister was wanted for murder at the time of the shooting. He struggled with alcohol, having been charged twice with public intoxication.

Fits Profile   Fatal   >16   Post-Secret Service

This is a postscript to Jamar Siler, the last school shooter profiled by the author and one who fit the profile of prenatal exposure to alcohol.

The first edition of The Fatal Link was published in November, 2008. In April, 2009, WATE Channel 6 in Knoxville, TN reported:

It was clear to the court Siler suffers from a conduct disorder created by a well-documented abusive past. His attorney believes Siler might also be suffering from fetal alcohol syndrome. "As you heard the judge say, there are major failures on the part of DCS in Florida, DCS here in Tennessee. This is a classic case of someone who has fallen completely through the cracks all his life. He never had a chance since he was a child."

This is the first time in the history of school shootings that an attorney for a school shooter has made any public announcement regarding the link between the shooter and prenatal exposure to alcohol. This announcement came five months after "The Fatal Link" revealed the connection between school shooters and their mother's drinking patterns.

Minnesota and Wisconsin Shooters not in Secret Service Study

25. Black, David, 15, Grand Rapids, MN, October 5, 1966

Fits Profile   Fatal   <16   Post-Secret Service   Confirmed heavy exposure

26. Anderson, Dicky, 14, Tomah, WI, Nov. 19, 1969
   Fits Profile   Fatal   <16   Confirmed heavy exposure

27. McLaughlin, Jason, 15, Cold Spring, MN, Sept. 24, 2003
   Fits Profile   Fatal   <16   Post-Secret Service   Mother denied exposure to alcohol

28. Wiesse, Jeff, 16, Red Lake, MN, March 21, 2005
   Fits Profile   Fatal   >16   Post-Secret Service   Confirmed heavy exposure

29. Hainstock, Eric, 15, Cazinovia, WI, Sept. 29, 2006
   Fits Profile   Fatal   <16   Post-Secret Service   Confirmed heavy exposure

Addendum Two of Two

The Mystery Man

In a small house in southern Louisiana, a baby boy was born. His father had died two months before he came into this world. His mother carried him, her third son, to full term. She had already been divorced once and had a son from her first marriage. This child was her third child, her second son with her now deceased, husband. Her second son later reported she told her children they were a burden to her and she sent her two oldest sons away to boarding schools. Neither of the older two boys had any reported behaviors.

His mother lived an itinerant lifestyle and before the age of eighteen, this young man had lived in twenty-two different residences and attended twelve different schools. During that time, his mother married again and the divorce records from her third marriage revealed she had a practice of throwing bottles at her husband when angry. He struggled in school and was placed in juvenile settings for truancy. Once, in a fit of rage, he attacked his mother with a knife. Another time, he attacked his brother with a knife.

He was arrested for truancy at the age of thirteen. While he was in juvenile hall, the adults who worked with him and examined him documented their belief that he had a quality about him that led him to act with an apparent disregard for consequences. His probation officer observed that he was "somewhat shallow, seemed to be immature, and have little capacity for comprehension." He told his Probation Officer he didn't like school, it was too hard, and he was not able to do the work. He also said he had too much difficulty making friends and liked to be by himself. A psychologist stated he, "had to be diagnosed as "personality pattern disturbance with schizoid features and passive aggressive tendencies." He also stated this young boy "has to be seen as an emotionally, quite disturbed youngster." The psychiatrist summarized his observations stating this thirteen year old had a "vivid fantasy life, turning around the topics of omnipotence and power, through which he tries to compensate for his present shortcomings and frustrations."

An official from the Salvation Army indicated that the boy, as pointed out in the psychiatric report, was severely disturbed and would need direct psychiatric treatment in a Child Guidance Institution.

A social worker concluded that this boy "just felt that his mother never gave a damn for him. He always felt like a burden that she simply just had to tolerate." He confirmed some of those observations by saying that he felt almost as if there were a veil between him and other people through which they could not reach him, but that he preferred the veil to remain intact. He admitted to fantasies about being powerful and sometimes hurting and killing people, but refused to elaborate on them. He took the position that such matters were his own business.

As this troubled boy grew into manhood, he began developing unrealistic fantasies of his place in the world. He joined the Marines and was dishonorably discharged. He acted on these fantasies of greatness and found disappointment at every turn. He married and soon after fathering a child, started abusing his spouse.

His writing and spelling was less than adequate, but he had the gift of gab, an ability to hold a conversation if he was talking about his fantasy world. People close to him continually found themselves struck by his lack of logic, remembering the young man's emotional inability to connect with potential friends.

He could not keep a job for any length of time. His employers found him to have poor people skills and a lack of employable skills. His world was crumbling around him as he continued fixating on his fantasy.

Let's examine his history. His behaviors clearly place him in the high probability of prenatal exposure to alcohol. His early pictures, including pictures of him when he was sixteen years old, reveal a thin upper lip and indistinct philtrum, distinctly different than his full blood brother. Using FASD 4-Digit Diagnostic Code and Lip-Philtrum Guides developed by the Washington State FAS Diagnostic and Prevention Network to make a comparison of his upper lip and philtrum using pictures available on the web, the argument can be made he has physical characteristics of FASD.

The mystery man's mother was of French and German descent and was a practicing Lutheran, a denomination and ethnic background that condones and celebrates drinking alcohol. Behaviors of his mother suggest she drank alcohol. She smoked. The testimony in the divorce proceedings of her third marriage states she threw bottles at her husband. Testimony revealed she was at least a social drinker later in life. The mystery man himself complained about his wife, saying she was too much like her mother. His wife liked to drink beer and sherry.

His older brother stated, when asked about his mother, "If we go and get right down to the bottom line, we have to say, really and truly, in all candor, she did a lousy job, a lousy job. By age three, he had the sense that his mother wanted to be someplace else. Mother would be putting him with a nanny, or a babysitter, or in an orphan home with us, just to get us out of her hair. We were a burden."

His full blood brother did not deny that his mother drank alcohol. I had sent him a letter with my findings and asked him for an interview. When I talked to him, he chose to not comment. He would not have known if or how much his mother drank when pregnant with his brother, as he was only a couple of years older than the mystery man.

Most significantly of all, his mother suffered a traumatic event seven months into the pregnancy, the death of her husband. It can't be confirmed, but this author believes the shock of her husband's death caused her to drink alcohol during that time at a rate much greater than before or after as a way of self-medicating to mask the pain. As a result of this binge of drinking during her pregnancy, her son had lifelong brain damage.

The probability of this mystery man entering this world as a victim of prenatal exposure to alcohol is very high. He had an unrealistic view of the United State's place in the world, and, because a friend of his wife found him a job in a building located near the route of the president, he impulsively took it upon himself to kill the leader of the free world to fulfill his fantasy of being someone. This mystery man was Lee Harvey Oswald.

For forty plus years, controversy has swirled around the belief of a conspiracy. As I read the volumes of interviews and testimony on the assassination of President Kennedy, I became convinced the act was his alone, the act of a brain caught up in the Perfect Storm of prenatally alcohol exposed brain damage and grandiose opportunity.

LaVergne, TN USA
01 February 2010

171635LV00001B/7/P